Drop Up To 8 Pounds In 8 Days

Detox Diet Cleanse

Boost Your Metabolism And Remove Toxins That Lead To Weight Gain

Victoria V Forres

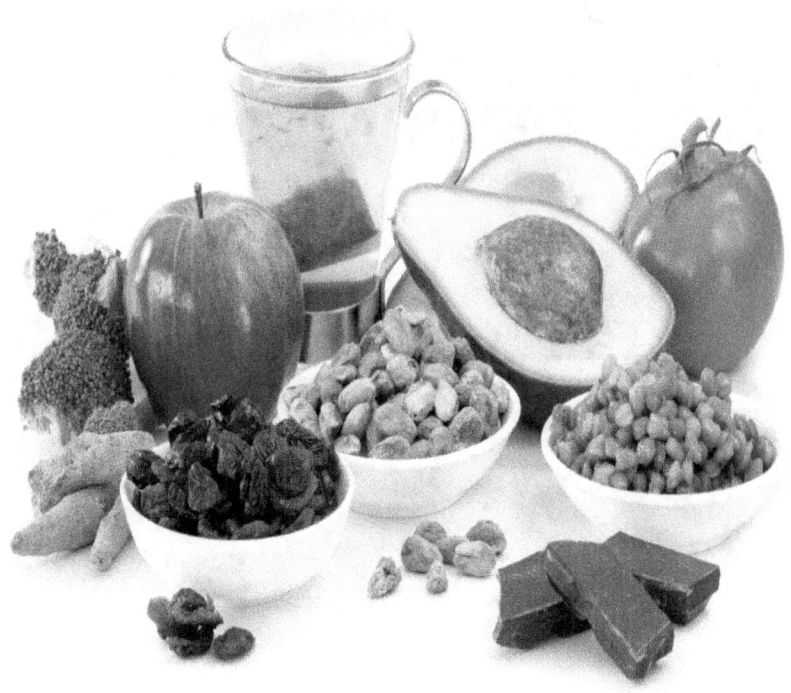

DEDICATION

To Harry, Nicole, Lewis, Jason and Douglas

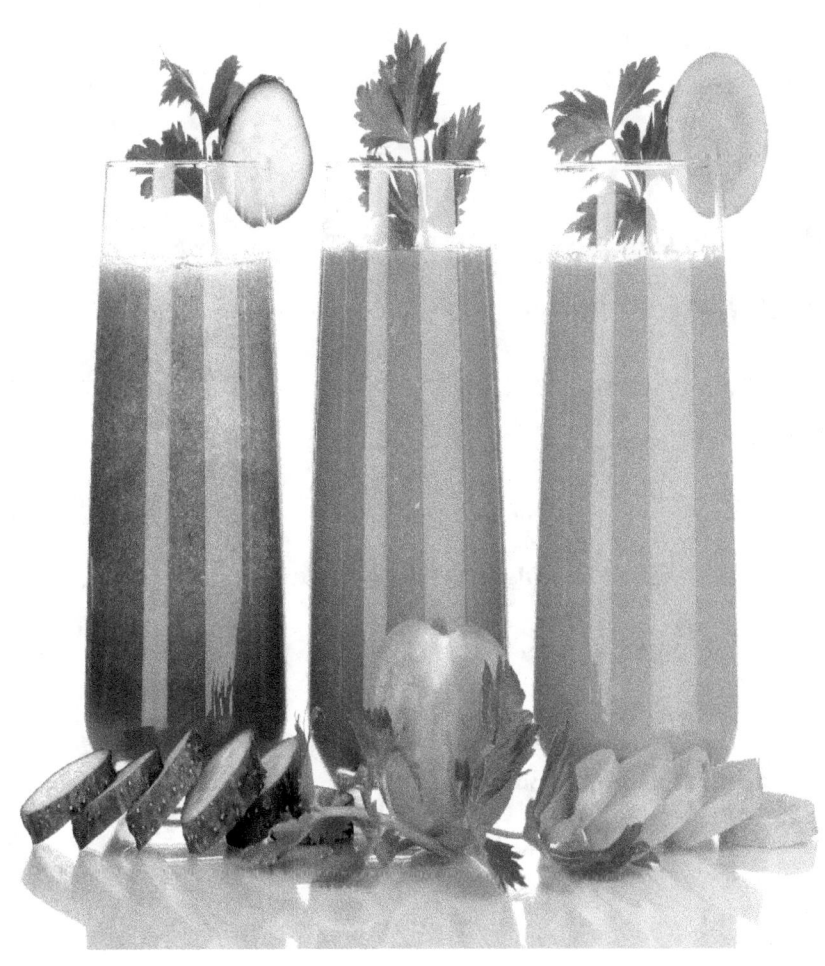

CONTENTS

Healthy Tips For During And After Your Fast Days iii

Weight Loss And Fiber v

Introduction 1

    How It All Began..1

    Crash Dieting...2

    Before You Start Any Dieting Program 5

History Of Vinegar 6

    Health Benefits Of Vinegar 8

    Vinegar Is Safe And Edible..9

    A Trusted Health Treatment..10

CHAPTER 1 11

    Apple Cider Vinegar Creation Process....................................11

CHAPTER 2 13

    How To Make Apple Cider Vinegar 13

CHAPTER 3 15

Cholesterol and Apple Cider Vinegar 15

Blood Cholesterol Levels 16

CHAPTER 4 17

Cholesterol Ratio And Apple Cider Vinegar...............17

CHAPTER 5 19

Honey And Apple Cider Vinegar Benefits...................19

Benefits of Honey with Apple Cider Vinegar 19

Benefits of Consuming Honey and Vinegar:...............20

Apple Cider Vinegar Health Benefits 21

CHAPTER 6 23

Honey Health Benefits 23

CHAPTER 7 25

Achieve Your Weight Loss Goal................................25

CHAPTER 8 27

Staying Healthy With Apple Cider Vinegar.................27

CHAPTER 9 29

Flavored Vinegars..29

How To Make Flavored Vinegar................................29

How To Use Flavored Vinegars 31

CHAPTER 10 33

Flavored Vinegar Recipes..33

CHAPTER 11 38

   Foods That Kills Belly Fat Fast 38

CHAPTER 12 43

   Be Watchful Where You Eat 43

CHAPTER 13 45

   Tips For Eating Out Healthily 45

CHAPTER 14 46

   Juice Fasting Detox and Cleansing 46

   Juicing for Healthy Living 47

   How To Choose A Good Juicer 49

   Different Types of Juicers 50

CHAPTER 15 52

   Juice Fasting And Weight Loss 52

   Cleansing Your Body Before Juicing 53

CHAPTER 16 55

   Benefits of Juicing 55

   Fruit And Vegetable Nutrition Benefits 56

CHAPTER 17 65

   Before You Start 65

   How Long Should My Juice Fast Last 65

   Long Term Fasting 67

CHAPTER 18 68

How To Break A Juice Fast...................................68

Breakfast 69

Early Morning Treats 70

Lunch 71

Afternoon Treats...72

Dinner 73

Night Treats 74

CHAPTER 19 78

Detox Recipes 78

Tomato Juice Detox...79

Nutmeg Elixir 81

Rhubarb Juice 83

Strawberry Kiwi Juice 84

Watercress Cleanse 85

Guava Juice Glory..87

Fruity Fennel Juice...88

Broccoli Sunrise 90

Lime Detox 92

Asparagus Juice Detox 94

Apple And Cucumber Detox 96

Ginger Root Delight..98

Celery Juice Detox..100

Kale Morning Glory..102

Sweet Morning Mango Juice................................104

Watermelon Juice Cleanse................................106

Cucumber And Carrot Juice................................108

Cabbage Juice..110

Blueberry And Cantaloupe Juice................................112

Sweet Radish Juice..114

CHAPTER 20..117

Weight Loss Juicing Recipes..117

BEFORE YOU START..118

Energy Rush..119

Parsnip Juice..120

Iron Boost..121

Celery Burst Juice..122

Grapefruit Punch Juice..123

Vitality Boost Juice..124

On The Go..125

Metabolism Boost Juice..126

Jalapeno Spice Juice..127

Green Rocket 128

Bumpy Ride 129

Cool Ginger 130

Pineapple Flush 131

Easy Lettuce Juice 132

Garlic Glory 133

Moody Blues 134

Cool Down Juice 136

Sleep Tight 138

Celtuce Juice 139

Loosen Up Chili Juice 141

Cantaloupe Juice 143

Flat Abs 145

Tangy Zucchini Juice 147

Refreshing Beet juice 149

Sweet And Sour Mix 150

Sweet And Sour Blues 152

The Lemon Mix 154

Vegetable Blues 156

Easy Going 158

Afternoon Glory 160

Refreshing Eggplant Juice 162

From The Author To The Reader 164

Conclusion 166

ABOUT THE AUTHOR 168

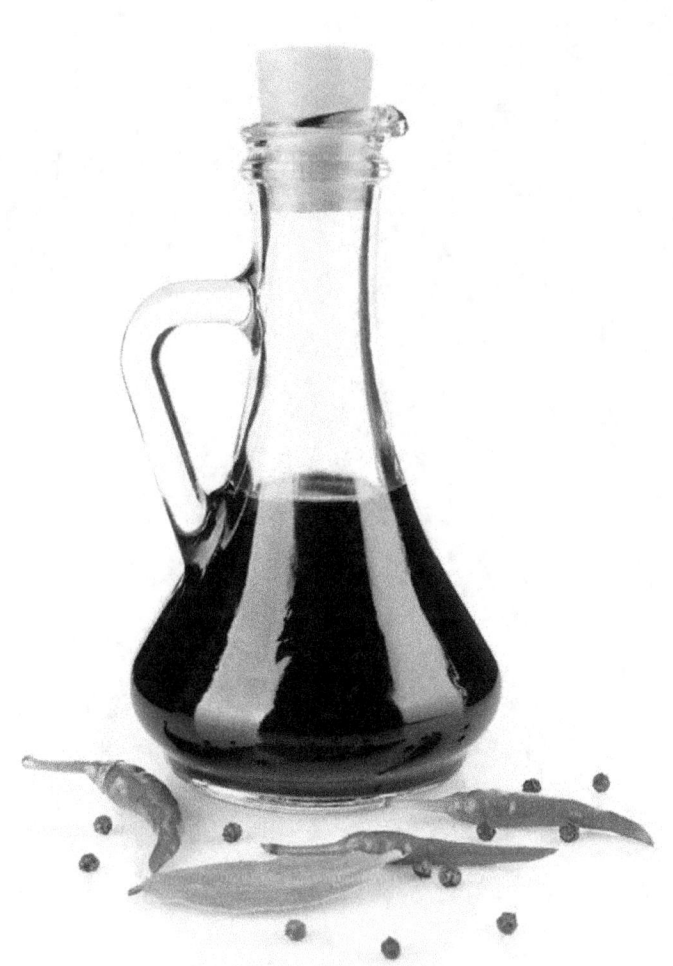

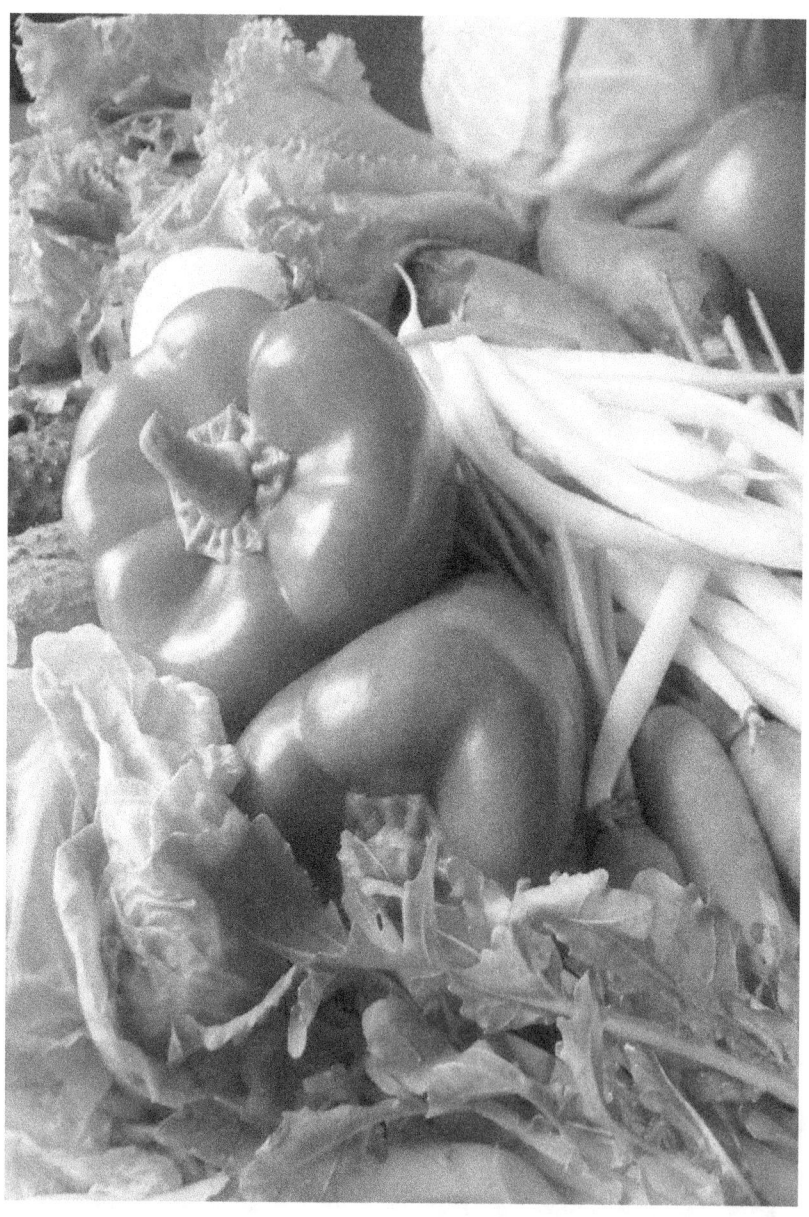

ACKNOWLEDGMENTS

I would like to thank Clark Wright, Paul Anderson, Scott Lee, Mark Harris, Carol Johnson, Barbara Levy, Jennifer Cowen, Laura Mitchell and Anthony Taylor, as well as the health care professionals who helped me on my journey.

✂ Drop Up To 8 Pounds

Detox Diet Cleanse

Healthy Tips For During And After Your Fast Days

☞ On your fasting days, avoid a lot of exercise. Consuming less food will make you feel a little weaker, to begin with, so don't put the pressure on yourself to exercise.

☞ Do not drink alcoholic beverage on your fasting days. Not only is alcohol packed with calories, it can also have a greater impact on your body than normal as you haven't eaten as much.

☞ **Don't quit!** Stay with it, even if you find your fasting days difficult to begin with, stick with it. **Remember!** You will soon be able to fit into your (goal) jeans and dress size and in a few days without having to feel guilty.

☞ Drink plenty of water during the day. It's good for you, has no calories, and can fill you up and help to stop cravings.

☞ When you are eating each meal, put your fork down between bites - it will make you eat more slowly and you'll feel fuller on less food.

☞ Drink a glass of water before and with your meal. This can help you feel fuller.

☞ Brush your teeth right after your meal to dissuade yourself from eating more.

☞ **See yourself thin!** Think of your goals and what you are trying to accomplish and stick with it. Remember you will soon fit into your dream dress or jeans.

☞ Acknowledge them, then distract yourself, if food cravings do strike. Take a long walk in the park or on the beach if you happen to live near one, phone a buddy, do a little gardening, or treat yourself at the spa.

☞ Whenever hunger strike, try waiting for at least 20 minutes and ride out the cravings. You'll find they pass and you can proceed with your daily activities.

☞ Feeling hungry is not a terrible thing. We're all accustomed to functioning on the smallest hunger pangs that we forget sometimes what it's like to feel genuinely hungry. Feeling hungry for a few days a week will not do you any harm. Learn to control **"hunger"** and take control of how you cope with it.

☞ **Get support!** Ask a friend or companion to join you on the Diet Cleanse. If you feel you can't do it on your own. Having another person to speak to can be very helpful and rewarding.

☞ Get moving. Being active isn't a necessity for the Detox Diet Cleanse to get results but as with all diets increased activity will help your weight loss efforts. Keep in mind what you're doing each day -- walk to the store instead of driving, instead of the elevator take the stairs.

Making small adjustments will not only help you burn off calories but can also give you more control of your weight loss and make you feel healthier.

Weight Loss And Fiber

Eating Fiber On A Daily Base Can

Help You Achieve Your Weight Loss Goals

Indeed, it is said that a "well-balanced diet" that is high in fiber, around 20 to 37 grams daily, is effective in the promotion of weight loss as well as maintaining a healthy and balanced weight. Which means! Your weight loss goals can be accomplished by increasing your day-to-day fiber intake.

A basic knowledge of the benefits of fiber along with the understanding as to how to get sufficient amount of fiber into the diet will help you to achieve your weight loss goals fast and in the most effective way.

There are a lot of factors as to why a diet that is high in fiber helps in the promotion of a healthier weight loss. Listed below are proven factors regarding why the intake of fiber is good for weight management:

Consuming Foods That are High in Fiber

Feeling fuller for longer is a good thing! Foods that are high in fiber makes you feel fuller for a considerably longer time. Foods which are higher in fiber give less calories per servings which makes you feel fuller for longer without having to eat as much. Fiber slows down the rate of digestion and stays in your stomach for longer, making you feel fuller for longer. High fiber foods usually require you to chew longer. This allows the individual to eat slowly, therefore making sure your body registers when it feels full sooner.

Fiber Is Not Easily Digested

This doesn't mean you will experience any fat gain by consuming high fiber meals even though you'll feel fuller. Fiber does not absorbed, nor easily digested by the human body. As a matter of fact, majority of your fiber intake is discharge from the body.

High Fiber Meals Are Normally Healthier

High fiber meals are usually better and healthier for you, because it is low in calories and full of nutrients when compared with other foods. Foods that's high in fiber makes you feel fuller without having to have an immense quantity of calories.

How many calories do I burn on a daily base? Good question! High fiber meals such as: fruits, legumes, lentils, vegetables, whole grains together with other legumes, are all recommended as a method of preserving and maintaining a healthful weight, and to keep the human body healthy.
It is relatively simple and easy to improve your fiber intake on a daily basis: on a daily base, consume 5 portions of vegetables and fruit.

Fruits that are rich in fiber include: bananas, apples, strawberries, citrus fruits, tangerines, prunes and pears.

✓ Add to your shopping list: whole-wheat pasta as an alternative for regular pasta, and brown rice as a substitute for white rice.

✓ For breakfast, go for high fiber cereals, like oatmeal or All Bran,.

✓ Eat whole-wheat or wholegrain bread instead of white bread which is low in fiber.

✓ In your daily diet, increase your intake of lentils, beans, as well as other pulses

Nibble on wholegrain snacks which are high in fiber, instead of chocolate.

The primary key to weight loss goals is to make sure that you lose a higher amount of calories than you consume on a normal basis. Eating a well-balanced diet which is high in fiber and doing regular exercise will guarantee that you shed that added weight quickly and successfully.

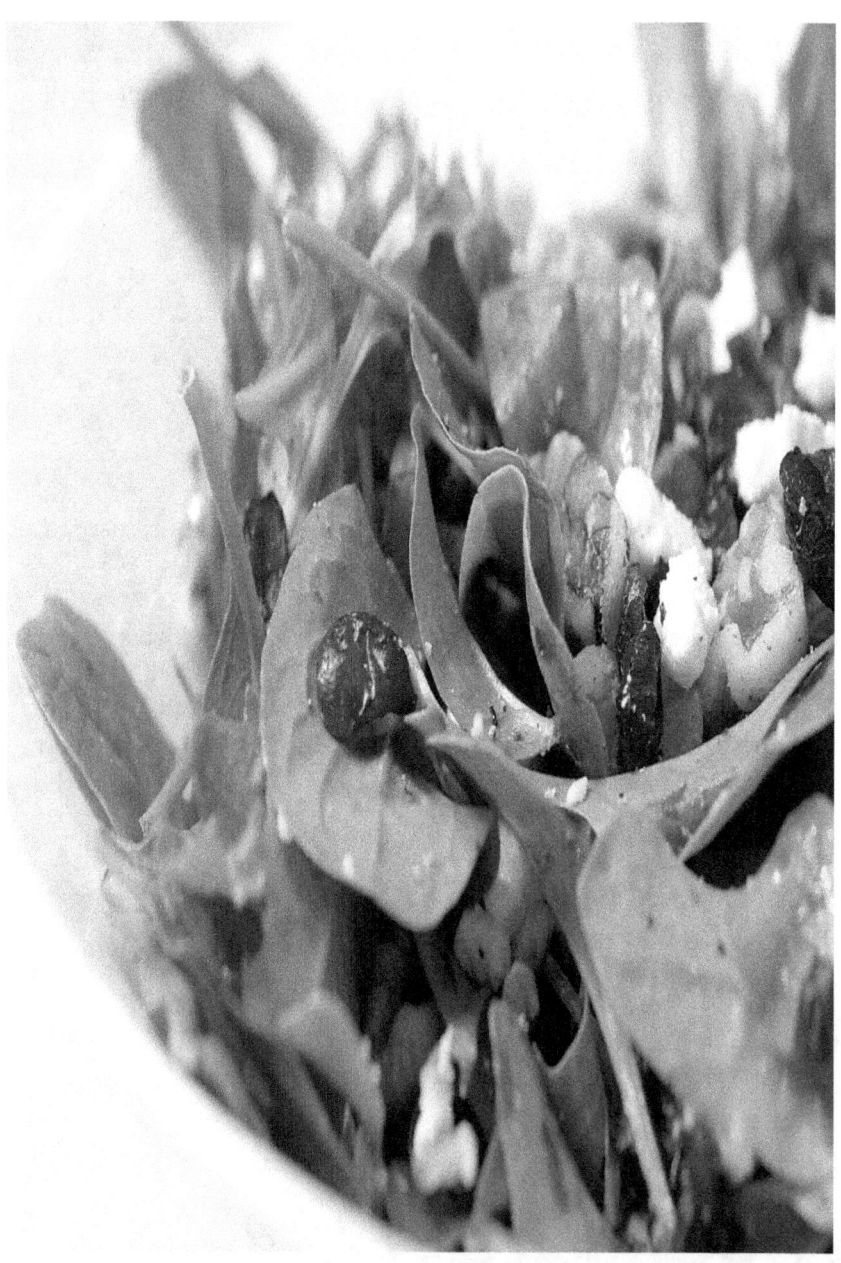

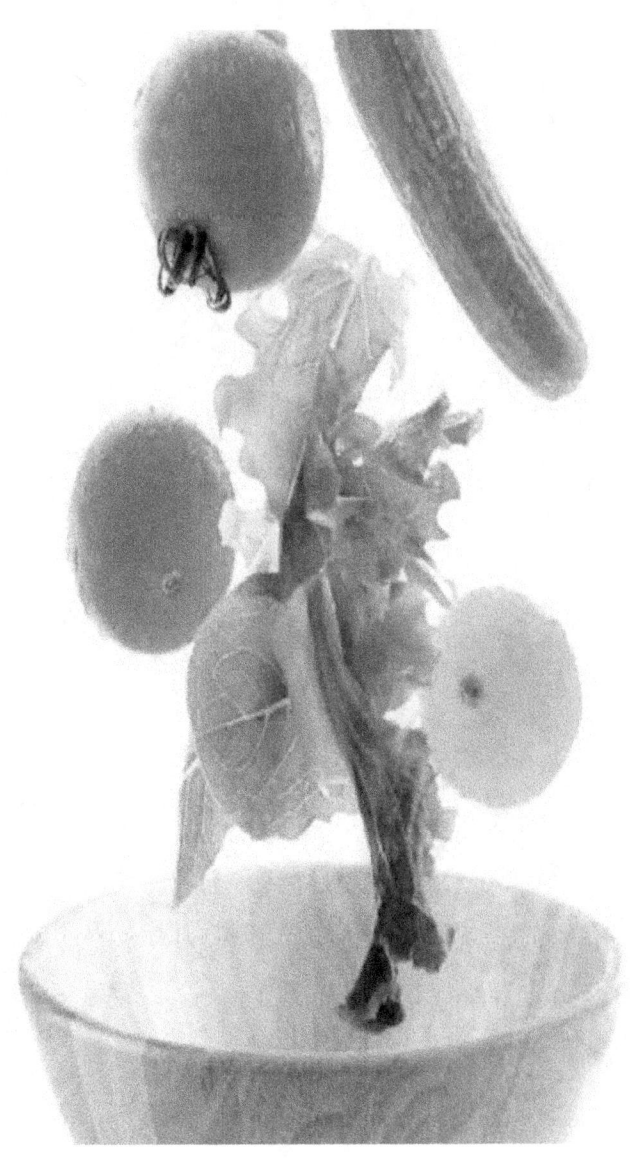

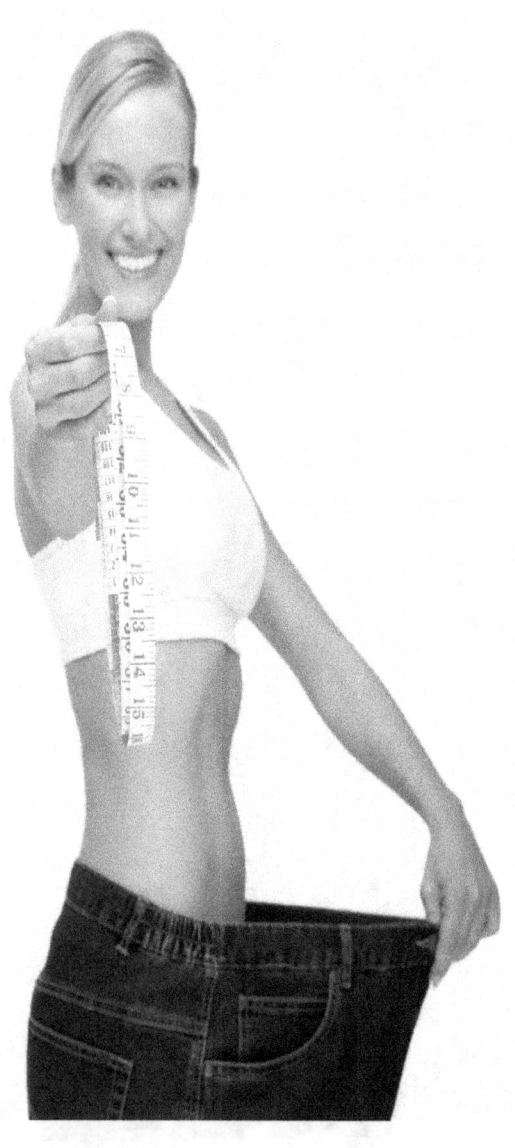

Introduction

I struggled all my life with my weight, I've been called many horrible names, and I had to pay extra for my size in clothing, because I was **THAT-- BIG GIRL**. I eat food for comfort and cried because I didn't fit in with the rest, I didn't have a man in my life for years! Why I hear you ask, "because I didn't feel comfortable in my own skin." Until one day it hit me! I began my journey with natural weight loss using "Vinegar Juice Detox".

How It All Began

My friend Nicole came to visit me 12 years ago and my life has never been the same. Nicole was that "BIG GIRL", depressed and sad. When she first arrived at my home, I looked her up and down --- I was astonished, and immediately noticed something was different about her; yes! the excess weight was gone.

I could hardly recognized her. But it was not just the weight loss that made her unrecognizable. She was happy, confident and looking radiant. I had to asked....how did you manage to lose so much weight? She said "Juice fasting and a little exercising."

I did not waste any time, I rushed to the store and bought all the green produce and fruits I could, because I was desperate for a change; not just to look better in clothing, but to be healthier.

Crash Dieting

Let's talk a little about "Crash Dieting" There's a saying that goes, if something seems too good to be true, then it usually is. Moreover, nearly all of those quick weight loss programs never live up to what they promise.

Oftentimes, crash dieting, or starvation diet plans as they're occasionally referred to, do nothing more than dehydrate the dieter, which means the amount of weight lost is called water weight. Obviously, the lost weight is gained back as fast as it was lost once the program ends.

Don't forget also that whenever someone goes on a diet, it means they'll likely come off it as soon as the goal weight is reached. But to maintain and keep a healthy weight means making lifestyle changes.

With fast diet plans you might lose a few pounds in a week or two and oftentimes days, you'll become a little slimmer, but most of the fat will remain, ready and waiting to take over the body once again.

There are still some things that you need to understand about these kinds of diets, even if this seems fine for all those peoples desiring to lose weight before a vacation, or some important occasion. The crash diet is one of the worst and most dangerous methods of losing weight period. In fact, it could result in direct harm to your physical body and affect your mood.

Yet despite this, these potentially dangerous eating plans continue to be legally encouraged all over, taking advantage of the vulnerable. In my personal experience, most weight-watchers that attempted to fight the excess weight have tried the fast dieting method at least once. But I also know individuals who go on these starvation diets frequently, and that's just asking for trouble since it's dangerous for the heart.

A recent study states that trying a crash diet once will not necessary harm your heart or your overall health. However, if you make it into a habit then you are putting yourself at risk, the chances of heart attack increases each time you go on a superfast weight loss programs. I always raised my eyebrows whenever I hear someone boosting how they have lost ten lbs in one-week.

Sure, they may have accomplished this, but keep in mind that 75per cent of our body is made up of water, and most of this quick weight reduction would have been exactly that - water. There's little point in shedding water weight if the fat still remains.

First thing that happens when on a crash diet is that you're eliminating muscle mass, and not fat, and less muscle means more fat. The repercussion of this is if you lose a lot of muscle you'll also lower your chance of losing weight.

After a few days on the crash diet you step on the scale and you see a lower number, right? This lower number is mainly a loss in water. The minute you come off your diet and start eating frequently again and hydrating, the weight will come back as fast, if not quicker than it went.

Another danger with fast weight-loss plans - when done too frequently - is the potential risk of organ damage. They can become stressed and inflamed, which consequently could make you more receptive to disease and more exposed to illnesses and catching viruses in general.

Furthermore, fast weight loss could adversely influence the way you feel and function as an individual. You ought to know also that individuals who embrace crash diets not only have the potential to gain extra weight after they quit following this insanity, but they're left having an insatiable craving because of their regularly unhealthy dishes, consisting primarily of fattening and processed food, which are also damaging to health.

I understand the minute an individual has chosen to take action regarding their weight; they want to see fast results. I also understand that a lot of peoples would like to get rid of these pounds with the least amount of discomfort and effort. It is essential to recognize though that there's no magic answer or quick-fixes; this just isn't the way that it works.

Losing weight does not have to be a lesson in pain, giving the dieter approaches it with the right mindset. If a person can accept that he/she need to put the work in (which includes a bit of perspiration), then you'll have a better chance of keeping a healthy and balanced weight, rather than gaining more pounds and putting your health at risks.

In this book I will show you how to lose weight and keep it off naturally; using "Vinegar Juice Detox" It is tried and tested! An old century remedy I've done it, Nicole has done it and you can too! **Are you ready to LOSE WEIGHT and feel great?**

Before You Start Any Dieting Program

Having the ability to speak with your family doctor concerning losing weight is a crucial thing; however it might be hard at times. You may have tried quite a few different exercise plans that didn't work out, and this could be because you didn't have the benefit of a medical expert's advice. It's better to ask for a doctor's guidance before you start any weight loss program.

The first doctor's visit is one of the most vital parts of your weight management program. The doctor will likely carry out a complete physical exam and blood work. This will determine if you have any underlying health problems which may be causing weight gain or the inability to lose weight.

After ruling out any underlying conditions, your doctor may go over physical exercise plans that work for you personally. When speaking to your doctor concerning weight loss, you need to be open and sincere. If there are conditions that may be creating issues with your weight loss goals, your doctor can treat and effectively address those.

Depending on your goals, your doctor may suggest different procedures. Generally, the doctor will gauge your level of readiness as your plan goes on. Doctors can assist with customizing exercise plans according to your health condition.

Speaking with your doctor is a fantastic way to get things on track from a physical standpoint. So your first assignment is to start speaking to your doctor about weight loss, and ensure your journey starts in the best possible way.

History Of Vinegar

The "Father of Medicine', Hippocrates (460-370 BC) is known to have recommended vinegar to his patients in order to renew the four humors into a balanced harmony. They were also the first to flavor vinegar with spices and herbs.

Apple cider vinegar originates from apple cider. The cider is fermented into alcohol, and the alcohol is allowed to continue fermenting until it becomes vinegar. All vinegar is created in this way; if you allowed your wine in your cupboard to continue fermenting, in the course of time, you'd have vinegar.

For centuries, apple cider vinegar is prescribed as a miracle remedy to treat all types of ailments - some cured, some not - and together with the resurgence of naturopathy in recent years, the vinegar has found itself back within the health limelight.

What can this unbelievable vinegar do to help you? In an environment of growing obesity rates, the most prized property of apple-cider vinegar is the way it can suppress appetite.

A recent research found a positive correlation between the amount of vinegar consumed and appetite suppression. Apple cider vinegar is prized for a completely different motive - it's shown to reduce blood sugar.

One study demonstrated that type-2 diabetics (without insulin shots) who took only two tablespoons of vinegar before going to bed were discovered to get far more stable levels of blood sugar each day.

Apple-cider vinegar is an inexpensive; all natural therapy that's virtually sure to enhance your wellbeing, should you endure type-2 diabetes, pre-diabetes or weight - associated insulin resistance, apple-cider vinegar is an inexpensive, all natural treatment that is sure to better your health. Studies also have discovered that vinegar can ease hypertension and lower cholesterol. It's really not yet known whether these same effects will be seen in human.

One study has demonstrated that individuals who consume vinegar based salad dressing at least five times weekly were at a significantly reduced risk of cardiovascular disease.

Further study will probably be necessary to nail the precise connection between cardiovascular disease and apple-cider vinegar; however, these early results are exceptionally promising.

Health Benefits Of Vinegar

Prior to the developments in modern medicine, vinegar, being accessible to the overall population, was utilized as a curative in many ways. It was-and still is-the foundation for many home remedies.

One could challenge most of the curative remedies credited to vinegar nevertheless vinegar certainly has properties which have helped in many different circumstances.

There are claims that vinegar can reduce osteoporosis, lengthen life, treat arthritis and dementia, and enhance hearing, eyesight and mental powers. There are still lots of ways that vinegar can be healthful both internally and externally, while all this could be well beyond its reasonable qualities.

All of the health benefits linked to vinegar is associated with cider vinegar made from apple cider or a base of processed apple parts. ACV has the same advantages of other vinegars and differs only because it is created from the juice pressed from apples.

Cider vinegar is the most common in America due to the abundance and accessibility of apples. Hard cider (historically a home-made, American alcoholic drink) upsurge to the normal utilization of cider vinegar.

Natural apple-cider that you just see within the health-food store isn't processed in the same manner, and that's the reason you'll generally find sediment in the bottom of these bottles.

Vinegar Is Safe And Edible

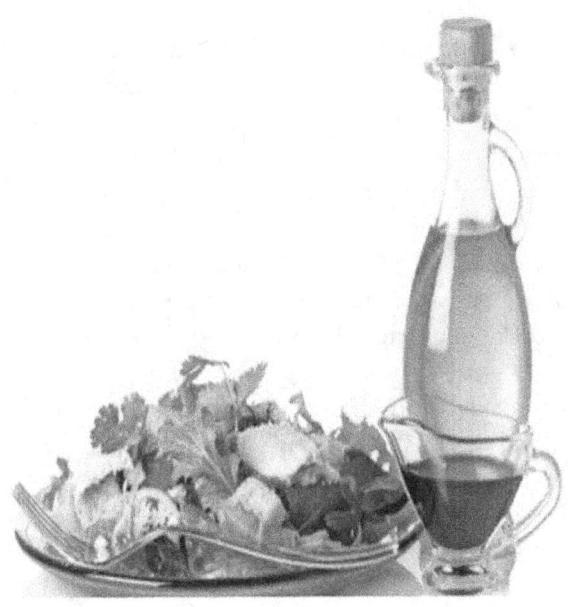

Vinegar is safe and edible, and it cannot hurt your stomach when ingested in small quantities. Multiple sorts and flavors of vinegars are available, in regards to food enhancements and vinaigrettes.

The world of culinary vinegars is a big one. Many types of vinegar are flavored by the addition of herbs or fruits; raspberry vinegar is one of the very popular. For the diet conscious, vinegar is fat free and low in sodium.

A Trusted Health Treatment

Vinegar has been a kitchen staple for a number of generations. It is really a trusted health treatment, a cleaner, a neutralizer, a condiment along with a preservative. Its acetic value permits it to eliminate germs, mold and bacteria while being secure enough to not harm the body or the environmental surroundings.

50 grains is the same as a 5% acid level, and it is probably the most frequent percent. Since distilled white vinegar isn't registered as a pesticide the label cannot claim it as a disinfectant.

Vinegar is available in higher acetic concentrations; however this is not easy to find in consumer shops as it can be more risky and needs to be handled with suitable precautions.

Use basic white distilled vinegar when a sharp acidity is preferred without the other features. Its nutrients are destroyed by the distilling process, making it a purer and much sharper acetic acid and clear in color. Many types of vinegar in stores today also have preservatives added.

Malt vinegars and brown rice vinegars are most frequently used in combination with "fish recipes." Distilled vinegar used for making pickles functions best with at least a 5% or higher acidity level. Always read the label carefully. In case it says wine vinegar, then it is vinegar, not wine.

Asian supermarkets generally carry three basic types of rice vinegar - black, red and white. As rice (the base) features a taste rice vinegars are normally milder.

The popular flavored rice vinegars have a mixture of sweeteners and salt added giving it a light taste. It has turned into a healthy option for all, like a salad dressing plus a flavor enhancer.

CHAPTER 1

Apple Cider Vinegar Creation Process

Beer vinegar and wine is among the many favorite foods that are manufactured by yeasts and microorganisms. The majority of vinegar starts as fruit juice which is exposed first to yeasts, and then bacteria, which work on fresh fruit sugars. At first these sugars are fermented by yeast to make alcohol.

Unique microorganisms breakdown the alcohol to create acetic acid, the main element in vinegar. Both bacteria and yeasts that produce vinegar are rich in nature, therefore when juice are extracted from the fruits, the liquids normally advance through stages of fermenting, after that vinegar is formed.

The natural inclination of juice to ferment describes why alcohol and vinegar are staples within the diets of virtually every culture around the globe since before recorded background. The word vinegar comes from the term "vinaigrette," or otherwise called sour wine. You can produce Vinegar from any fruit.

You may have seen a thick, opalescent substance floating near the top of any organic vinegar. This substance is called "the mother." It contains cellulose that results from the interaction of the bacteria with the alcohol. In some cases the mother of vinegar is believed to be accountable for the creation of vinegar. Acetobacters is a bacteria which is responsible for the conversion of alcohol into vinegar.

Acetobacters need oxygen as a way to develop and survive. If alcohols like apple cider are exposed in open air for a few minutes, the interaction of the acetobacters and oxygen while in the air helps with the transformation of alcohol into vinegar. It can be used to introduce these organisms into cider, since the "mother" of vinegar will have a concentration of acetobacters clinging to it.

The type of the bacteria is somewhat mystical. The alcoholic content falls and the level of acidity rises, as cider is transformed into vinegar. The easiest way to know whether the process is complete is by tasting it; no odor or flavor of alcoholic beverages should exist.

The effectiveness of the vinegar depends upon the quantity of alcohol in the cider. The vinegar for home cooking is approximately 4 to 6% acidity. Therefore the alcohol level of the apple cider vinegar must be about the same percent.

CHAPTER 2

How To Make Apple Cider Vinegar

You can buy some amazing all-natural apple cider vinegar in health shops; however it's a lot more satisfying creating your own. Fill a broad mouthed jar about two thirds with apple cider, If you'd like to make your own vinegar from cider.

Add to the cider either a tiny amount of unpasteurized, unfiltered all-natural apple cider vinegar or some mother of vinegar accessible at some health-food shops or where brewing ingredients can be bought.

Cover the top with cheesecloth, so the bacteria from the vinegar will have access to air without being contaminated by bugs. Place the jar in a dark room at room temperature for four weeks. The best way to know if the vinegar is ready is by tasting it, this is the best process method which was applied for years and years.

There must be no further taste of alcoholic, after the vinegar is ready. For those who have a "wine examining kit", you'll be able to test the vinegar until it's about five or six percent acidity. This straightforward homemade procedure was most likely the first way vinegar was produced.

And there was more interest in industrial production, manufacturers developed a way using wooden barrels filled halfway with wine and laid on the sides as the use of acetum became more popular.

This strategy is frequently referred to as the field process or Orleans process for the French town where this technique was most notably employed. Using the barrels on their sides, as opposed to upright, more surface area of the wine was exposed to the air.

The well-known French scientist Pasteur, who wrote numerous reports on the bacteriological processes involved in making vinegar, was instrumental in devising a type of wood "raft" that would float at the top of vinegar barrels and help keep the "mother" together with the vinegar. Time is also an important variable in making tasty and flavorful vinegar; much the same way as aging makes excellent cheese or wine.

To speed up the process, holes were often pierced at either end of the barrels and coated with fine mesh screen to help keep out contaminants. Various other techniques were created where wine or cider was passed through a tank filled with wood chips, charcoal, as well as corn cobs to raise the surface that came in connection with the air, to shorten the time needed for fermenting.

Throughout fermentation, especially during commercial production where high quality vinegar is produced, it is essential not to interrupt the vinegar in progress. If the "mother" of vinegar which usually floats on the surface is moved, it may sink to the bottom of the container and decompose, detrimentally impacting the flavor and quality of the vinegar.

CHAPTER 3

Cholesterol and Apple Cider Vinegar

Some level of cholesterol has to preserve the healthiness of the cells in the body and to also create hormones secretions that activate different organs and glands. There are two kinds of Cholesterol, good cholesterol and bad cholesterol. Cholesterol is a waxy metabolite that exists in the blood

HDL - high-density lipoprotein is called 'good cholesterol' and the human body is expected to increase the percentage of HDL in the body as much as possible. HDL helps eliminate the unwanted (poor) cholesterol from the walls of the blood vessels.

LDL-CHOLESTEROL or Low density lipoprotein is called 'unhealthy cholesterol'; it is responsible for making a soft, oily, wax-like plaque in the internal walls of the blood vessels.

Accretion of LDL in arteries can obstruct the vessels and may lead to inadequate stockpile of blood towards one's heart or brain. This problem can result in a heart-attack or even a stroke. Liver creates the required amount of cholesterol.

Apple cider vinegar helps the liver to maintain a regular flow of blood, and cleanse the body of toxins. For this reason, the vinegar will help to improve the function of the liver.

Blood Cholesterol Levels

Our physical body gets cholesterol from the food that we eat. In fact, cholesterol created by the liver is sufficient for the requirement of the body and we need not have it from outside. HDL needs to be above 60 mg/dL. HDL less than 40 mg/dL substantially increases the danger of cardiovascular disease as well as stroke.

LDL ought to be less than ONE HUNDRED mg/dL. LDL 130 - 159 mg/dL is considered as 'borderline high' and more than 190 mg/dL is taken into consideration as 'very high'. Overall cholesterol needs to be less than 200 mg/dL.

The ratio for ldl/hdl must be generally higher than 0.4; however any ratio above 0.3 is thought to be inside the usual levels of cholesterol range.

if you're thinking of trying apple cider vinegar for reducing the blood cholesterol, you could regulate this ratio, as it would allow you to understand if consuming vinegar has effectively worked for you or not. Reducing cholesterol levels without medication is possible, if you follow the information on reducing cholesterol.

Try to Include low fat dairy products in your diet on a daily base, eat good fats in the precise proportions, avoid high fat meat (have lean meat instead) and deep-fried foods. Staying clear of cholesterol rich meals such as egg yolk can assist in the prevention of high blood cholesterol

CHAPTER 4

Cholesterol Ratio And Apple Cider Vinegar

Consuming Apple cider vinegar to reduce high cholesterol is an olden holistic treatment. Ayurveda doctors from ancient Egyptians and ancient India have announced endless benefits of the apple cider vinegar. They've used it habitually to treat sicknesses of all sorts, as they understood that it increased the flow of blood circulation to the body.

Most vinegar begins as fruit juice which is exposed first to yeasts, then bacteria, which work on fruit sugars in different ways. Initially these sugars are fermented by yeast to create alcohol. Then specific bacteria break down the alcohol to form acetic acid, the main component in vinegar.

Both the yeasts and bacteria that make vinegar are plentiful in nature, so after the juices are extracted from the fruits, these liquids naturally progress through stages of fermentation, then acidification.

The vinegar dissolves mucous secretion, fat, cholesterol, arterial and joint deposits; that may cause serious health problems. Therefore, 'apple cider vinegar for high cholesterol' has become the essential phrase, when exploring the solutions to manage cholesterol.

By making dietary adjustments, it is possible to lessen as much as 30 percent of unnecessary cholesterol. Low cholesterol diet which includes foods that lower cholesterol normally is the best method to regulate blood cholesterol levels.

One tbsp. of Apple cider vinegar with a small amount of honey to add taste if taken every day, works great for blood cholesterol. You can use Apple cider vinegar instead of white vinegar when cooking, as it makes no distinction in taste.

Your cholesterol count will be within a healthful and protected range again. Vinegar also helps you to shed pounds naturally and alleviates joint pain. Apple cider vinegar contributes to several roles when included in regular diet and helps improve your health and well-being in different ways.

Apple pectin, a water soluble dietary fiber existing within the apple-cider vinegar, consumes the fat molecules and unhealthy cholesterol. It boosts excretion of those unwanted substances and minimizes their levels. Liver plays an essential part within the metabolic processes, as you probably already know.

If the ingested food is not metabolized correctly, it contributes to 'weight gain'. Vinegar enhances the process of digestion of fatty meals. It can help speed up the metabolic rate of fats, proteins along with other elements present in food.

This way, it encourages weight loss. Therefore, health and wellness benefits of the Apple cider vinegar are of great importance. So, among each of the natural treatments, apple-cider vinegar is the number one choice.

CHAPTER 5

Honey And Apple Cider Vinegar Benefits

A mixture prepared from honey and apple-cider vinegar has been utilized for an exceedingly long time to treat several illnesses, especially pain in the joint. Even though this is actually the biggest perk of regularly drinking a glass of honey mixed with water and apple cider vinegar, you will find many other advantages of the two when consume on a regular base.

Whether on their own or together, apple cider vinegar and honey are beneficial for your body. Below, we have a look at apple cider vinegar and honey when mixed together and how it can be helpful to the body.

Benefits of Honey with Apple Cider Vinegar

When taken together, honey and apple cider vinegar has great benefits to our health. Vinegar is a naturally acidic product, however, if consumed; it turns alkaline in the body.

The essence of the alkaline from the vinegar has made it an excellent treatment to respond to the ill-effects of a highly acidic diet that we eat in regards to fast food and so forth.

Furthermore, it is well-known to be used as an important treatment for pain in the joint and arthritis. Honey gives a similar result when used as treatment as well. Though it has a reduced pH, it becomes alkaline as soon as it is consumed, and assists in the safe excretion of high levels of acids in the entire body.

Honey is normally added to apple-cider vinegar to ensure it is simple and easier to consume by toning down the sharp taste of the vinegar.

Even after that, you may not find the drink to be delicious. However, when you begin, you will want to keep consuming it on a regular basis, because of the adjustments you will start to experience within your body. A few of the perks you are likely to experience by drinking this mixture are given below.

Benefits of Consuming Honey and Vinegar:

- Relief from indigestion or constipation

- Relief from joint pains

- Removal of halitosis (bad breath)

- Relief from sore throat

- Delayed aging process

- Reduced cholesterol levels and blood pressure

- Boosted stamina and energy levels

- Relief from pyrosis (heartburn)

- Weight loss

Apple Cider Vinegar Health Benefits

- Apple cider vinegar helps with the treatment of sinus infection and clears sore throat.

- It helps in stabilizing the cholesterol levels.

- In regards to treating skin problems like acne, few come close the effectiveness of apple cider vinegar.

- Additionally, it shields us against most forms of gastrointestinal disorder.

- Apple cider vinegar assists in curbing allergic reactions in animals and humans.

- It reinforces our defense mechanisms and prevents muscle weakness after exercise.

- Vinegar raises the entire body's metabolism which encourages weight reduction, eliminates constipation and enhances digestion.

- A mix of lecithin and vitamin B6, and apple cider vinegar is thought to be among the best dietary medications for weight-loss.

- It relieves the pain from arthritis and gout.

- Its consumption prevents bladder stone and urinary tract infections.

- Vinegar has acidic properties, which is used for treatment for bad breath.

- The sulfur in apple cider vinegar , helps to fights aging process. Thus, it's used as a treatment for liver spots.

- It is used by women as a treatment to reduced cellulite.

- It's also used for as a treatment for serious ailments such as hypertension and diabetes.

CHAPTER 6

Honey Health Benefits

Honey is among the best treatments for arthritis. For treating arthritis, Combine and make a mixture of one teaspoon cinnamon powder, two parts lukewarm water and one part honey. Apply the mixture to the joints which is most distressing; this will lessen the pain in fifteen minutes.

Vinegar is also used for treating hair thinning and baldness. Before having a bath, prepare a mixture one tablespoon of honey, one tablespoon warm olive-oil, as well as a teaspoon of cinnamon powder, and apply the mixture on your scalp leave on for a few minutes.

Honey is also an effective treatment for toothache. Prepare a mixture containing five teaspoons of honey and one teaspoon of cinnamon powder, and apply it directly on the aching tooth.

Honey is quite effective, when it comes to lowering cholesterol. To lower cholesterol, make a combination of honey, cinnamon powder and 16 ounces of green tea. Drinking this mixture will lower the cholesterol level instantly.

It is quite powerful against acute coryza (common cold). Combine one tablespoon of honey with 1/4 tbsp. of cinnamon powder. Have this for three days; this will undoubtedly get rid of the cold. Honey combined with cinnamon powder also helps in reducing stomach ache.

For weight loss, prepare a concoction of honey with cinnamon powder and water, and consume it on a daily basis. This helps decrease the buildup of fats.

CHAPTER 7

Achieve Your Weight Loss Goal

TASTY HONEY COCKTAIL AND APPLE CIDER VINEGAR TO LOSE WEIGHT

All the previously mentioned advantages of honey and apple cider vinegar are obtained when consumed in their raw and natural forms. Refined variations of both offer small nutrients, and might not hold the same advantages as stated previously.

Bear in mind that all-natural products will probably be higher-priced in stores. To determine whether it is organic or not, you could examine the label and the product appearance. When compared to the processed counterpart, all-Natural honey or apple cider vinegar is often cloudy.

To prepare this drink, mix together:

1 teaspoon, Raw Apple Cider Vinegar
1 teaspoon, Raw Honey
8 oz. Warm Water

Drink at least two times daily on an empty stomach. Some beneficiaries of the beverage may recommend drinking this up to four times daily.

This will depend on how much of the drink you can consume due to the strong taste of the vinegar. If you want to experience the benefits of this drink you must at least try it for a couple of weeks.

CHAPTER 8

Staying Healthy With Apple Cider Vinegar

Can eating an apple a day really keep the doctor away? It can certainly help you to control your blood sugar and gain all the benefits that come with that control. In fact, researchers have found that women who eat at least one apple a day are 28 per cent less likely to develop 'Type 2 diabetes compared to those who do not eat apples.

That is probably because apples are filled with soluble fiber - the number one for blunting blood sugar level swings. A medium apple serves up an outstanding 4g of fiber, mainly pectin, which is known for its capability to reduced cholesterol.

Planning to get rid of your belly fat? (Keep in mind, stomach fat is bad for blood sugar.) Try eating three small apples each day.

A recent report from the State University of Rio de Janeiro discovered that doing so as part of a reduced-calorie diet plan not only assisted women to shed more weight but additionally helped them to reduce their blood sugar levels significantly more than women who ate another food as opposed to apples.

To get every little benefit from apples, go for whole, unpeeled good fresh fruit. The apples with the lowest GL are Brae-burns, which have more acid and not as much sugar than Golden Delicious.

Following on the scale is unsweetened apple sauce, which offers several of the exact same health and wellness benefits. However, stay away from apple juice; it's not much better than apple-flavored liquid sugar.

Like many fruits, apples include vitamins, minerals along with other antioxidant properties which may help decrease the chance of cancer by preventing DNA damage.

Boron, the mineral that is found in apples, may possibly retard bone loss in women after menopause and may help women on estrogen replacement therapy keep the estrogen in their system for much longer.

Using a suitable mix of mindful eating, plentiful exercise and apple-cider vinegar, your weight loss goals can be reachable. Remain focused, and have patience - all it takes is a little bit of dedication. Calorie counting and exercise alone will not take off fat, but apple cider vinegar is a crucial element to make the process painless.

Not only will your blood sugar stabilize as well as your blood pressure lowered, but the appetite suppression properties of apple cider vinegar will protect you from your hunger pangs that plague most dieting hopefuls. Regardless of your goal, if you have 10 pounds to lose or 100 apple-cider vinegar will help. Your health will enhance, and your energy will grow.

CHAPTER 9

Flavored Vinegars

Lately there's been a burst of flavored vinegars available in the market. Particularly with balsamic vinegar of which there are currently varieties featuring herbs and flowers.

Although considered as wine vinegar, it is in fact generated from grape pressings that haven't been permitted to ferment into wine. It's rich, smooth depth of taste is imparted to the food when used in cooking.

How To Make Flavored Vinegar

Creating your own flavored vinegar is easy. White vinegar is frequently used as a base, because its clarity and high acid content will complement the variety of added ingredients. Rice vinegar and apple cider vinegars are often used as well. You may use leaves of herbs or sprigs, hot peppers, raw garlic to create your own flavors.

If you choose to use fruits like raspberries, it is essential that you first cook down the fruit adding a tbsp. of honey or sugar to the mixture before pouring it into a wide mouth jar of your choice and then cover it with vinegar.

Cool, cap and label, and give it a week or two before tasting. Flavored vinegars should last no less than 2 years when stored in a cool dry area. Berry fruits can alter color but they do not spoil as the vinegar is a safe preservative.

- Make your very own hot vinegars by carefully warming 1qt of vinegar to which you've added dry spices such as cinnamon sticks, peppercorns or whole cloves. Wait until the vinegar is cooled then strain, bottle and label.

- Put your peeled cloves of garlic from a whole garlic bulb in a quart glass jar. Fill it with white vinegar or white wine vinegar and let this sit covered tightly for at least 2 weeks.

If you only have a metal jar lid, put a small plastic sandwich bag underneath the lid so the vinegar will not come in contact with it. It will have a powerful garlic taste. One teaspoon garlic powder will replace for 1 garlic clove.

- Lavender vinegar is created with unseasoned rice vinegar using a few sprigs of lavender, left to stand, and covered, for a couple of weeks. This type of vinegar is not for contributing to food but to utilize as a warm fragrant, deodorizer or cleaning product.

- Sterilize new containers that you're using for flavored vinegars to stop the vinegars from clouding.

- Make your own portion of wine vinegar by adding a tablespoon of white or red wine to two tablespoons of white vinegar. If you desire to make a larger amount use 1/4 to 1/2 cup of red or white wine to 1 cup of white vinegar or cider vinegar.

- Use rose petals or any sweet smelling flower to give a

wonderful aroma to some white vinegar.

How To Use Flavored Vinegars

➢ Make a fast vegetable or cracker dip by combining 4 tablespoons mayo with 1 teaspoon of your flavored vinegar of choice.

➢ Save the juice from fish cooked in vinegar and add a little to some basic vinaigrette. Use it on the salad you serve with the fish for a complementary taste.

➢ Add a touch of any herb flavored vinegar when making tuna salad.

➢ Give a new flavor to your favorite potato salad recipe calling for white vinegar by using an herb flavored or seasoned rice one in its place.

➢ Make marinated mushrooms that have been rinsed and stems trimmed by first bringing them to a boil and simmering in a sauce pan for 10 minutes: 3/4 cup vegetable or olive oil, 1/2 cup of an herb flavored vinegar, 1 teaspoon salt, 1 teaspoon sugar, 1 bay leaf and a few peppercorns.

Put in one pound or so of mushrooms and simmer for 3 minutes uncovered. Put mushrooms and fluid into a pan. Cover and cool for several hours or overnight. Remove bay leaf and peppercorns and drain mushrooms.

CHAPTER 10

Flavored Vinegar Recipes

Rosemary Vinegar

Makes 2 cups

One pound of fresh rosemary sprigs. Two cups white wine or cider vinegar.

This recipe can be used with many different herbs - try using:

• thyme
• tarragon
• bay
• marjoram

The more delicate herbs for example basil, dill, coriander and mint will need their leaves bruising a little. Avoid using dried herbs or spices since these could make the vinegar cloudy for maximum flavor.

- Remove the woody stems from the rosemary and place half in a glass bowl. Pour over the vinegar, stir and then cover lightly, leave in a cool area for 7 days stirring occasionally.

- Strain, discarding the rosemary. Repeat with all the remaining rosemary and pour the strained vinegar over. Cover lightly and stir occasionally afterward leave for a further 7 days. Add 2-3 rinsed sprigs of fresh rosemary and screw down tightly.

Keep in a dark place.

Spiced Vinegar

Makes 4 pints/3 cups

6 tsps. peppercorns
3 tsps. mustard seeds
2 tsps. allspice
1 blade mace
1 large cinnamon stick, bruised
4 fresh bay leaves
1 small piece of root ginger. Chopped
1 tbsp. salt
3 cups malt vinegar

This is ideal if you desire to make your own chutneys and pickles, You can alter the spices used according to your preferred taste, White distilled vinegar is frequently used since it provides a sharper tang, however white wine, red or malt vinegar is great to use too.

Tie all of the spices into a piece of muslin cloth and place in a nonreactive saucepan. Add 1 cup of the Vinegar and bring to the boil. Boil for 3 minutes then add the remaining Vinegar and boil for a further 3 minutes. Remove from the heat and leave covered for at least 24 hours. Strain into sterilized bottles and screw down.

Raspberry Vinegar

Perfect for mixed greens or fruit salads
Bruise 1 cup fresh raspberries and put them in a sanitized vessel.

> Heat wine vinegar or white to below the boiling point.
> Pour the vinegar in the vessel and cover tightly.

Leave for two to three weeks.

Lemon Thyme Vinegar

> Peel one lemon in a thin spiral (removing the colored part only) and put in a sanitized jar with four to five springs of lemon thyme or thyme.

> Heat the white vinegar below boiling point.

> Pour vinegar in a jar and cover tightly.

Leave for three to four weeks.

Remove peel and thyme then Strain vinegar. Put the vinegar in a clean jar, adding peel and fresh thyme sprigs for garnish. Seal tightly.

Orange Mint Vinegar

Use in dressing for tossed green salads with orange and grapefruit sections or in marinades for chicken or lamb chops.

- Peel one medium orange in a very thin spiral (removing the colored part only) and put in a sanitized jar.

- Gentle bruise 1/2 cup freshly mints leaves and add to jar.
- Heat white vinegar or apple cider to below boiling point.

- Pour the vinegar into a jar and cover tightly.

Leave for three to four weeks. Remove mint and peel then strain vinegar. Put the vinegar in a clean jar, adding peel and fresh mint for garnish. Cover tightly.

Basil Garlic Vinegar

Use in dressings for rice, pasta, antipasto salads or in flavored mayonnaise.

- Put 1/2 teacup crudely cut fresh basil leaves and two cloves of garlic, peeled and split, in a sanitized jar.

- Heat white vinegar or wine vinegar boiling point.

- Fill the jar with vinegar and cover tightly.

Leave for three to four weeks. Uncap, strain vinegar and discard garlic and basil. Put the vinegar into a sterilized jar; add a little fresh basil to garnish. Cover tightly.

CHAPTER 11

Foods That Kills Belly Fat Fast

HOW TO HAVE A
HEALTHY LIFESTYLE

It is really no secret that veggies and fruits are good for you. You probably already know a few of the health benefits, including lower blood pressure and reduced danger of diabetes, cardiovascular disease, stroke and certain cancers.

You might even understand that eating fresh fruits and vegetables may lower your chance of losing your eyesight as you get older. Yes, vegetables and fruits are rich in vitamins, a large number of fiber and health protective compounds.

But are you aware that consuming more of these is a vital strategy in losing weight and keeping it off? With the exception of a few starchy vegetables, a large proportion is quite low in calories.

That's because they're mostly made up of water and fiber (both of which have no calories). Studies show that the more vegetables and fruits people eat, the less they tend to weigh.

It truly can be as easy as eating a salad. In a single study at Pennsylvania State University, women who started a meal with a low-calorie salad and then ate a pasta dish had about 12% less calories altogether than women who started with the pasta and skipped the salad.

With some exceptions, there's absolutely no need to avoid this vegetable or that fruit since it contains sugar or will raise your blood sugar.

Most fruits and veggies are actually very low in total carbs and contain fiber - often the soluble fiber that slows blood sugar's rise - therefore their GLs are quite low. So don't hesitate to nosh on apples and pile your plate with vegetables.

Foiling High-GL Carbs

You'll reduce the GL of a typical portion of any carb dish by combining in nearly any vegetable or fruit (again, potatoes do not count). If you include spinach, carrots, and tomatoes to a pasta salad, for example, you'll eat less pasta.

Should you add chopped broccoli into a rice side-dish, you'll eat less rice; the same goes for adding strawberries to warm or cold cereal. And fewer carbohydrates equal lower blood sugar.

Let us consider a rice side-dish. A portion of 180g of cooked long-grain white rice has a GL of 23, which makes it a high-GL food.

However, equal weight of boiled dried peas has a GL of only 3, so in the event that you mix an equal number of peas using the rice, a 150g portion of the side dish could have a GL of only 13, changing it from a high- to a medium- GL food. Actually, combining any vegetable in your rice - chopped cooked onions or asparagus or carrots - likewise lowers its GL.

Snack

Whole fruit is always a great snack option. For example, a 50g pack of potato crisps has a GL of 14 - making it a medium-GL food (but only when you consume this much with no more).

However, a medium peach or plum has a GL of only 5, and the GL of a similar sized apple is 6. Additionally, you are consuming twice as much food; therefore which do you think will probably fill your hunger best? The GL would be just 16, even if you ate a peach, a plum and an apple.

On the flip side, in case you munched your way through 100g of crisps, the GL for your snack would be considered a much bigger 28. Raw vegetables are also Super snacks, dipped in low fat sour cream, low-fat dressing.

Pack a few cherry tomatoes or carrot sticks in a sandwich bag and you'll not have any reason to hit the vending-machine. Fill up on veggies of various colors, since various colors indicate different health protective compounds.

A Few Exceptions

Just about all fresh garden produce is beneficial to us, but specific kinds are not as beneficial to our blood sugar levels. When we mention to eat more veggies and fruits, we're referring to colorful vegetables (not starchy vegetables or potatoes) and fresh, whole fruit, whenever we tell you to consume more fruits and vegetables. Here's the lowdown:

Potatoes

These really are the exception: they are dense in easily absorbed carbohydrates, so their GL is fairly high. Actually, the more potatoes, including chips, that an individual eat, the higher their threat of diabetes.

Many dietitians believe potatoes ought to be labeled with grains rather than with veggies, and even then they are at the peak of the carbohydrate pyramid.

Other Starchy Vegetable

Winter squash and sweet potatoes are rich in carotenoids and other essential nutrients as well as fiber, which can be advantageous. Although their carbs aren't readily absorbed as those in white potatoes, they are also high in carbs.

That makes a much better alternative to them than white potatoes, as with several other carbohydrate - rich foods, keep an eye on your portion size.

Juices

By drinking only the juice, you'll pass up on all the fiber and a few of the vitamins in the entire fruit, and also you'll get much more calories along with an increased GL.

If you eat 125g of fresh pineapple, for example, the GL is 6. But should you really drink a little glass (180ml) of pineapple juice, the GL is 12.

The same goes for grapefruit (GL 3) versus a little glass of grapefruit juice (GL 7), and for orange (GL 5) versus a little glass of juice (GL 10). Also if you go for a Hugh sweetened fruit drink, the GL soars: a 375ml glass of cranberry juice cocktail has a GL of 36.So if you drink juices, be attentive to keep portions small, and also make certain they are unsweetened (read labels carefully).

Dried Fruits

Drying concentrates the sugars in fruit and will make for intensely calorific treats. It is good to get some raisins, dried dates, plums, figs and apricots, but do not overindulge in them.

Study what happens when plums (GL 5) turn into dehydrated prunes (GL 10) or grapes (GL 8) turn into raisins (GL 28). A handful, or 60g, of dried dates has a whopping GL of25.

CHAPTER 12

Be Watchful Where You Eat

Make the task of eating out easier by selecting carefully where you eat out. Prevent the temptation of all-you-can-eat places, or buffet-style restaurants, where portions are hard to control. Avoid places that are famous for their large portions.

And it's likely safe to say you will not find lots of super foods on the menu at eateries that specialize in deep-frying an entire breaded onion. Enjoy a meal at one of those on your birthday, for sure, but do not do it on a normal basis. Not if you desire to do your blood sugar and well-being a favor.

Order Creatively

Whenever you order, be daring: order soup or salad to begin with, instead of an entree; or carve an entree and share a side order of veggies to get more vegetables in your meal - and less calories. Ask if you're able to have an additional vegetable instead, if your main dish has a potato.

If you intend to order dessert, plan to share it, too. The most effective policy would be to really get to know the size of these portions as well as a restaurant, what they serve and also to utilize that information to make practical alternatives from the menu.

Make Friends with the Waiter

Get prepared to befriend the servers or waitresses, as soon as you're in the right kind of restaurant. Ask them to keep back the bread basket so you are not tempted to fill-up on usually high GL carbs while waiting for your meal to get arrive.

If it does not come automatically, ask for water when you sit down. Drinking water will help fill you up. Before you order, have a look across the restaurant to find out what others are ordering. If the portions are large then choose two starters or share a main course with a friend.

CHAPTER 13

Tips For Eating Out Healthily

It would be simple to eat out, if most restaurants offered menus filled with Super cuisine for example lean grilled meats, wholegrain side-dishes, and fruit-based desserts. However they don't. Almost all the most common carbohydrate-rich meals on menus represent those in the normal Western diet. In other words, they're high GL meals.

And at most restaurants, from fast-food joints to the fanciest white tablecloth establishments, the food is full of extra calories and floating in butter add to the Hugh portions that we've grown to anticipate for our money, and eating out seems impossible to do well.

However, it can be achieved and understanding how is a survival skill because we eat out - or have takeaway meals - so frequently now. Fifty years back, eating out was mainly a luxury; today, based on the Food Standards Agency, males eat a quarter of their everyday calories outside the home and women a fifth. The very first step will be to accept how generally you eat foods you have not made yourself, then plan to order better.

CHAPTER 14

Juice Fasting Detox and Cleansing

Juice fasts have become a popular treatment to help cut back on calories and fat, also to help individuals shed weight. Juice fasting, also called "juice cleanse," is a detoxification diet that will require the person to consume healthy juices to get nutrients. This fasting method is used by dieters to remove excess fat and toxins from the body while abstaining themselves from eating food completely.

Unlike diet plans based on controlling specific oily foods or needing the intake of nutritional supplements, juice fasts are a natural option to help the body lose extra weight. Encouraging the intake of healthy and balanced foods, Juice fasts nutritional supplement a low calorie diet with veggies, fruits and legumes that have liquids

Supplements as well as dietary plans can help in shedding weight successfully, yet they likewise can be damaging. The majority of diet plans are unsafe considering that they strip the physical body of important nutrients needed to burn fat.

Juicing for Healthy Living

Juicing boosts the entire body, it's delicious, a great way to give your taste buds a treat. Juicing is by far one of the quickest, most delicious and best ways to get all the daily vitamins and mineral your body needs.

A recent research shows that the healthiest foods for the body are those that are easily digested. Then this concept only stands to the reason that juicing is the most effective and the best way to obtain a healthy and balanced nutritional intake daily.

When fruits and vegetables are used in making juice, the vitamins and minerals found in them are preserved, and because there's little digestion required for all these nutrients, the effects are felt instantly throughout the body.

After drinking a glass of fresh and delicious juice your energy will increase, because the fruits and vegetables are all natural the body will quickly absorbed it.

In addition, your body will have the ability to get a concentrated amount of enzymes from the fruits and vegetables when used for juicing. The enzymes are quickly taken into the body and helps in the conversion of foods into energy and body tissue.

The more enzymes the body takes in, the more efficient your digestion is likely to be and therefore the more efficient your metabolic rate will be too.

This contributes to an enhanced digestive system, less fat buildup and more effective wastes removal process. Also consuming a fresh glass of fruits and vegetables consistently will guarantee that your body gets the correct amount of phyto-chemicals, which are essential components in the body's ability in combating illness and disorders.

With all the great things juicing has to offer, it should be part of your day-to-day lifestyle. Besides from the benefits of juicing, there are other things to know, such as, how to store your juice after juicing. Always remember that it's advisable to drink juice immediately because all the nutrients and enzymes are in their freshest and purest form.

How To Choose A Good Juicer

Juicing fresh fruits and vegetables on a daily base offers lots of health benefits. Juicing supply the body with vitamins, antioxidants, bioflavonoids, minerals, enzymes as well as other nutrients which's necessary to maintain and keep our bodies strong and healthy. However, to make this possible and less complicated for you, you need to have your own juicer.

Getting your own Juicer is a superb alternative to purchasing pricey juice drinks in the food stores that normally contain lots of sugar and preservatives. Having your own juicer allows you to make your own juice drinks, giving you the choice to tailor the flavor combinations ideal for you and your family members.

Different Types of Juicers

Centrifugal

The least expensive Juicer, centrifugal juicers are likewise the most preferred selection. They are ideal for individuals using a restricted budget. The centrifugal juicer includes a disk that spins the juice out, catching the leftover pulp in the basket.

Citrus

Marketed both as a manual and an electric model, this type of juicer is good for juicing citrus fruits.

Manual

With one of these you will need to use your muscles to squeeze out the juice on your own using cheesecloth to filter the pulp.

Masticating

Very popular and known for making juice without foam: This type of juicer is ideal for baby sauces, baby food, and sorbets.

Triturating

This type of juicer uses twin gears to shred and press the juice from the vegetables and fruits. Although more pricey than the other choices, triturating juicers extract more juice, which is better for you.

Wheatgrass

A great option to juice wheatgrass; a one of a kind feature that as a powerful motor. Juicing with a much more effective juicer is often quicker. Depending on the size of the individual home; cabinet space, kitchen counters and dimension will be one more thing to consider when shopping for a juicer.

Power and size

When you purchase a juicer with a robust motor, you will not need to chop fruits or veggies thoroughly. In addition, juicing with a more highly effective juicer is usually quicker.

CHAPTER 15

Juice Fasting And Weight Loss

Does Juice Fasting Help?

As one of the hottest crazes in the weight loss business, juice fasting is preferred for its ability to get rid of excess fatty tissues quickly. Yet, the question remains: does juice fasting help in regards to weight loss? **The answer is yes!**

For individuals who are planning to lose weight quickly, juice fasting will help in achieving fast weight loss goals. Individuals who've used this approach to lose weight have reported losing approximately one pound a day.

It's recommended to avoid foods that are rich in carbs after fasting, while juice fasting produces an excellent beginning to a weight loss regime. Juice fasting reduce calories in the body.

When using a juice cleanse, the body improves its absorption of nutrients since the colon walls become free from impacted feces. Going back to high-calorie enriched meals after fasting will only create weight gain instead of continuing loss.

Cleansing Your Body Before Juicing

Before you start any juice fast, make certain you cleanse your body a few days before. It's essential to ensure that you cut out all fatty foods and dairy products especially fast foods. All these are damaging to your quality of life including your body.

Stick to fish, vegetables and fruits; chicken is an excellent source of protein. Do this two days before you start your detox. This will help your body to become primed for the push in weight loss that's about to occur. Remove any sodas, sweets, sugary drinks, carbs and caffeine from your diet.

Once you experience the wonders of juicing and see the results, you will be astonished! Doing a juice cleanse is a way to remove toxins and build-ups from your body and still provide your body nutrients to absorb and function the way it should. You will lose sheets of fat and you will become strong and happier.

Toxins can build up in our system and impact us in many different ways. You may experience these signs if you have a buildup of toxins in your body:

- Constipation
- Tissue Inflammation
- Headaches and Overall Lethargy (laziness)
- Multiple Allergies

During a juice cleanse you may experience one of these symptoms:

- ➢ Weakness
- ➢ Fatigue
- ➢ Increased moodiness
- ➢ Nausea
- ➢ Sore muscles

Should you experience any of these, don't panic, it's normal. This simple means the body is adapting, and is healing itself as well as rejuvenating. If the symptoms become life threatening or you feel they are beyond those listed here, you should stop the juice fast and speak with your doctor.

CHAPTER 16

Benefits of Juicing

Doing a juice fast has many proven benefits, which makes it a preferred way for people who desire to detoxify their bodies. The most preferable ingredients are all-natural vegetables and fruits, when deciding on a juice fast.

All-natural is effective and more suitable since one of the main goals of this particular method is to free your body of toxins. Although it might be hard for you to afford organic produce, try to buy the very best high quality you can afford.

Furthermore, there are some fruits and vegetables that are stronger than others. For example, try to purchase all-natural blueberries along with other berries, fruits including oranges, cukes, and pineapples are ones where you may remove their peelings before juicing.

Juice is high in nutritional content: Juice is a very natural source of water that's full of proteins, minerals, carbs and vitamins. Likewise, Juice is plentiful in essential fatty acids, bioflavonoids, enzymes, carotenes and chlorophyll.

These nutrients are in a form which our bodies can easily absorb, when consume in juices. All of the nourishment you get from juice is not usually found in foods we consume whole because cooking food can cause some nutrients to be lost during cooking.

For example, vitamins A, D, E, and K are water soluble vitamins which are prone to heat. Juicing helps maintain and preserve these minerals and vitamins because they're not heated. This results in sustained nourishment for the body.

Fruit And Vegetable Nutrition Benefits

Apple

Pectin, Boron, Cellulose

Reduces risk of Alzheimer's disease, detox liver, cataract prevention, neutralizes irritable bowel syndrome, reduces cholesterol and promotes a healthy heart.

Banana

Vitamin B6, Vitamin C, Anti-Oxidants, Copper, Magnesium

Helps depression, increases brain power, prevents weakening of bones, reduces ulcers, lowers blood pressure, menstrual pains and regulates bowel.

Beetroot

Calcium, Potassium, Folic Acid, Iron

Helps the digestive system and reduces high blood pressure, production of antibodies, natural mood lifter, detoxes the liver, antioxidant and good for immune system.

Blackberries

Niacin, Foliate, Vitamin A, C, E & K

Relieve PMT, reduces hot flushes, destroys free radicals, protects against heart disease, promotes production of blood cells and protects the skin from UV rays.

Broccoli

Folic Acid, Vitamin C, Beta Carotene, Calcium, Iron

Regulates blood pressure, eases cold symptoms, healthy nervous system, eye health, strengthens immune system and helps repair skin damage.

Cabbage

Calcium, Anti-Oxidants, Potassium

Maintains healthy and clear skin, helps eczema, relieves headaches, fights coughs and colds, helps fight osteoporosis, reduces blood pressure, and prevents arthritis.

Watermelon

Potassium, Vitamin A & C, Anti-Oxidants

Promotes weight loss, blood pressure , osteoporosis, immune system, erectile dysfunction, heart, eye health, blood pressure, kidneys, gout, heart and sex drive.

Collard Greens

Calcium, Foliate, Vitamin A, C & K

Boosts immune system, lowers cholesterol, protects against cancer, helps with menopause, protects against cataracts, antioxidant, aids in weight loss.

Coconut Water

Riboflavin, Calcium, Potassium, Iron

Regulates blood pressure and speeds up metabolism, aids weight loss, indigestion, balances electrolytes, anti-inflammatory properties, and boosts energy level.

Cucumber

Vitamin K, Prosperous, Potassium, Silica

Aids digestion, bad breath, controls blood pressure, promotes joint health, and stimulates hair growth, natural diuretic, Rehydration and glowing skin.

Cranberry

Vitamin C, E & K, Magnesium

Excellent anti-oxidant, help prevents plaque forming on teeth, maintain a healthy urinary tract, good for the eyes, heart, and reduce peptic ulcers.

Ginger

Manganese, Potassium, Magnesium, Vitamin B6

Morning sickness helps in the treatment of ovarian cancer, motion sickness, mood lifter, migraine relief, menstrual cramps, and cold and flu prevention.

Grapes

Copper, Iron, Magnesium, Anti-Oxidants, Vitamin C

Reduces cholesterol, migraine, help prevent heart attack, helps asthma, a natural diuretic, reduces blood pressure, anti-aging properties, and keeps you regular.

Honeydew melon

Vitamin A & C, Foliate, Niacin,

Boost immune system, anti-oxidant, sweet fix for weight loss and diabetics, glowing skin, and reduces blood pressure and good for pregnant women.

Strawberries

B complex, Anti-Oxidants, Niacin, Riboflavin, Vitamin C

Blood pressure, detoxifies, thyroid gland, immunity, liver, anti-inflammatory, eye health, brain health, gout, arthritis, anti-oxidant and heart.

Carrot

Fluorine, Vitamin A & C, Potassium, Anti-Oxidants, Pectin

Lowers risk of heart disease, slows down aging cells, helps maintain healthy eyes, healthy teeth and gums, cleans colon, glowing skin.

Kale Leaves

Calcium, Manganese, Iron, Anti-Oxidants, Vitamin A & C

Powerful anti-oxidant, detoxifying, Aids liver function, boosts nervous system, autoimmune disorders, essential to reproductive organs, fights against arthritis, asthma.

Kiwi Fruit

Anti-Oxidants, Potassium, Vitamin A, C E& K

Fights male impotence, cleans colon, protects eyes, good during pregnancy, and reduces the potential for blood clots, reduces respiratory disease.

Lemon

Ascorbic Acid, Calcium, Iron, Vitamin A, Prosperous, Copper, Potassium

Detoxifies, fights infection, relieves digestion problems and heart burn, reduces stress, liver cleanser, and assists with breathing problems and throat infections.

Mango

Vitamin A, C & E, Vitamin B6, Anti-Oxidants, Potassium, Magnesium

Supports eye health, great for skin, aids digestion, alkalizes body, remedy for heat exhaustion and anemia, beneficial during pregnancy, boost memory.

Mint Leaves

Vitamin A, C & E

Removes toxins, asthma, and diuretic, eases stomach pain, lessens symptoms of irritable bowel syndrome, and helps keep skin clear

Olives

Iron, Omega 9 B1 and 2, Vitamins A, C, DE & K

Anti-inflammatory properties, reduced hypertension, lower cholesterol, menopause, and antioxidant, helps ulcers, and contains good fats.

Celery

Potassium, Vitamin A, C & K, B1 and 6 Foliate

Lowers blood pressure, natural diuretic lowers cholesterol, anti-inflammatory properties, fighting bad breath and helps ease symptoms of a urinary tract infection.

Orange

Pectin, Potassium, Calcium, Vitamin C

Healthy skin, helps prevent kidney stones, Maintains healthy bones and teeth, improves sperm count, boost immunity, brain development and reduces arthritis pain.

Honey

Fructose, Glucose, Riboflavin, Iron

Reduces throat irritation, great for the skin, probiotic, mood enhancer, reduces acne, helps hangovers, aids sleeping and Increase athletic performance.

Pawpaw

B complex, Potassium, Vitamin A

Arthritis, aids blood clotting, prevents cramps, blood pressure, promotes fertility, strong bones, and glowing skin, helps prostrate and helps eyesight.

Tomato

Anti-oxidants, vitamin A & C, beta carotene

Gall bladder, hair, anti-oxidant, cholesterol, Kidney stones, hypertension, detoxify, prostrate, anti-inflammatory, vision, helps migraines and strengthen bones.

Lettuce

Vitamin C& K, Foliate, B-Complex, Magnesium, Iron

Heart disease, helps prevent insomnia, helps build blood cells, aids digestion, support nervous system, cleanser and reduces risk of cataracts.

Pear

B complex, Vitamin A & C, Anti-Oxidants

Throat problems, shortness of breath, reduce allergies, osteoporosis, Increase energy level, immunity, antioxidants, coughs and colds.

Pineapple

Potassium, Magnesium, Vitamin C, E & K

Blood clots, digestion, arthritis, sun stroke and blood clots, macular degeneration, helps sinusitis and bronchitis, good for gums, strengthen weak bones.

Prunes

Vitamin A & K, Vitamin B6, Riboflavin, Niacin

Gout, decreases cholesterol, bone density, bones, and anti-oxidants, slows aging process, blood pressure, and reduces stress.

Radish

Calcium, Vitamin C, Riboflavin, Thiamin

Colds and flu, anti-contestant, liver and gall bladder, fever, stomach, urinary tract conditions , digestion, skin, detoxifies blood , blood pressure and cholesterol.

Raspberry

Vitamin A, C & E, Beta Carotene, Foliate

Glowing skin, liver, anti-oxidant, burns fat, increases energy, antihistamine properties, arthritis, healthy colon, anti-viral properties and anti-inflammatory.

Spinach

Iron, Calcium, Vitamin C, Anti-Oxidants, Potassium

Increases energy, anemia, osteoporosis, eye health, gum health, bones, gastrointestinal health, strong teeth and Slows down aging process.

Parsley

Vitamin A & C, Anti-Oxidants, Folic Acid, Iron,

Anti-inflammatory properties, ear infections, strengthen bones, diuretic, upset stomach, keeps heart healthy, anemia and promotes wound healing.

CHAPTER 17

Before You Start

Keep in mind to peel off any hard skins and remove seeds before juicing. Wash all the fruits and vegetables thoroughly to get rid of any dirt and chemical residue. Drink your juice within ten minutes after juicing to keep all the fresh nutrients. You can also add a small amount of water -- mineral water and ice-cubes or crushed ice depending on your preference (you can try out all the recipes to match your very own necessities).

How Long Should My Juice Fast Last

Individuals diet for various reasons. A lot of people fast or diet as a means to shed excess weight and cleanse their bodies of toxins; while others fast for renewing their spiritual life. Every person is different, and our physical bodies work in different ways also.

The length of a juice fast can vary from one to sixty days. You should always start small, and then move up to longer days. Start your juice fast on a 3 day trial and break for a week. Then return for another 7 days.

A lengthy juice fast is more effective than a short one. Nonetheless, if it's your first time fasting, it is recommended to start with a fast that lasts 1 to 3 days so that the body can adjust to the whole process. As with all these health scenarios, it is important to listen to your body and know your limits.

Juice Fasting Is Not For Everyone!

Juice fasting is not right for everyone. It's necessary to get your physician's approval before you start. Despite the fact that juicing is safe and also a very effective and powerful method to lose weight, juice fasting isn't safe for people with illnesses like metabolic syndrome, diabetes, gout, pregnancy or during breastfeeding.

If you're uncertain, always talk with your doctor regarding this matter. You should begin with a one day then fast for three days-- slowly moving up to five days, once you've the all clear from your doctor. If you're trying juice fast for the first time and wish to do a five day trial; always start on the weekend.

This will give you a flexible schedule as you start to observe and understand how fasting works and the effects it has on the body. If you're encountering issues constantly stop immediately! Pay attention to what your body is telling you and you will know if you should carry on with the fasting.

You can try and stretch the length of fasting further-- to ten days, until you accomplish a thirty days juice fast, when you achieve an easy seven-day juice fast. You have already mastered some of the issues you might encounter through the initial day one or two, for example how to deal with hunger pangs. Longer juice fasting is actually possible, especially if you're used to fasting.

Long Term Fasting

Long term fasting can be beneficial to the body as it gets an uninterrupted period of cleansing, healing and repair. A lot of people who have tried lengthy fasting-- roughly between 30 to 40 days-- have seen several changes in their health.

These changes range from healthy weight loss, reduced water retention, increased emotional, psychological and spiritual sensitivity, increased and improved mental clarity, a Hugh boost in energy levels, cured allergies and many other health benefits.

CHAPTER 18

How To Break A Juice Fast

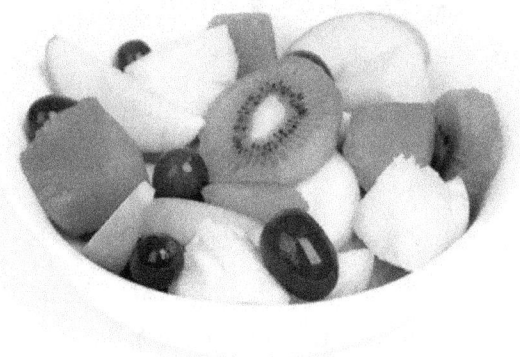

Breakfast

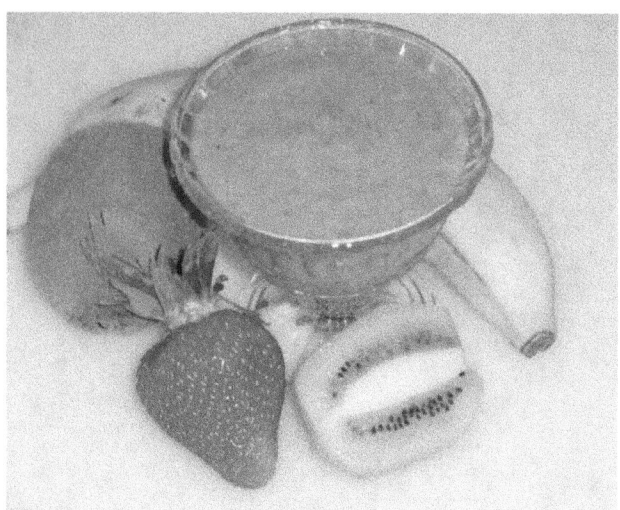

You can have a smoothie or fresh juice, a piece of fruit or a vegetable salad and a cup of herbal tea.

Early Morning Treats

You can choose any fresh juice.

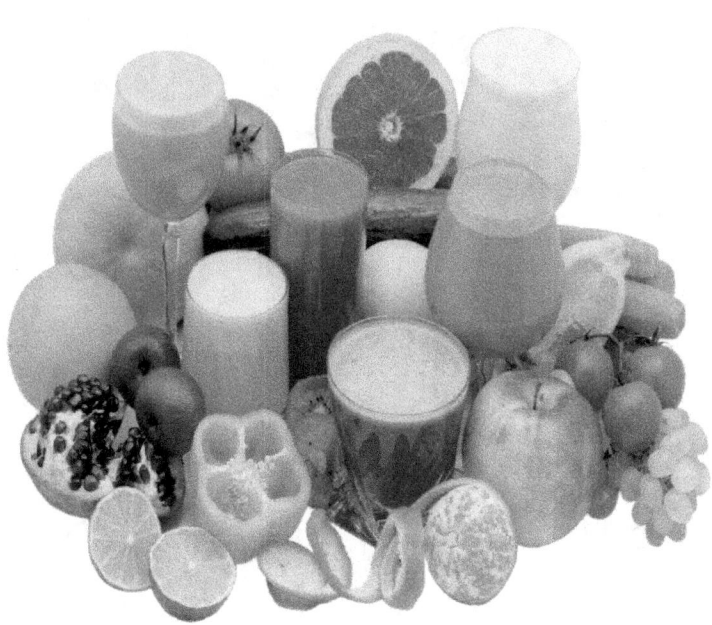

Lunch

A light vegetable soup with a salad

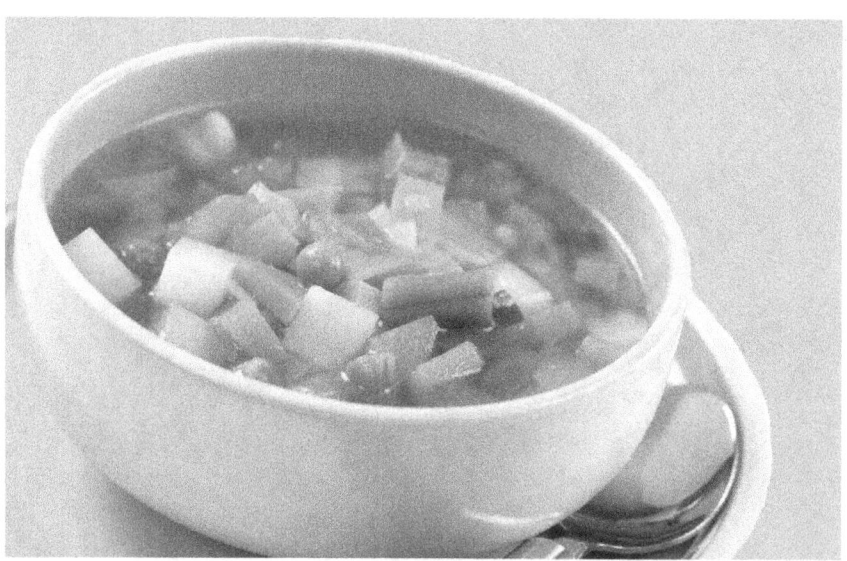

Afternoon Treats

A glass of: Any fresh juice of your choice.

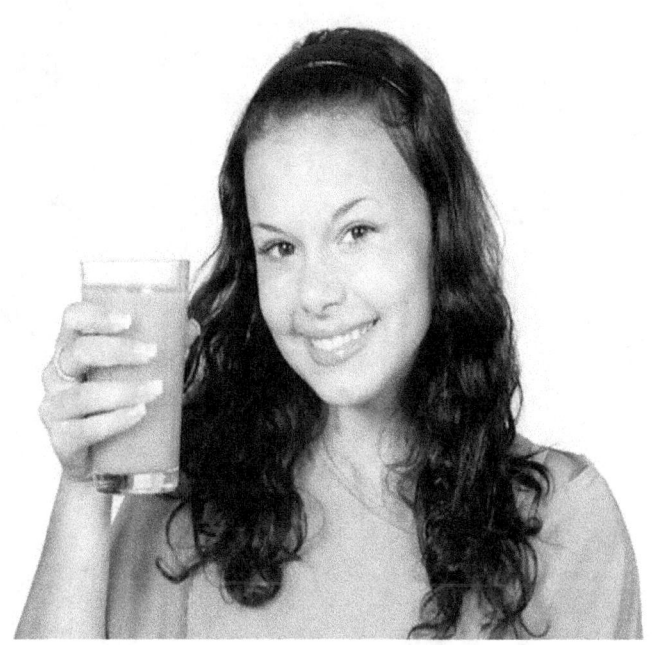

Dinner

A small bowl of: Lightly steamed vegetables, vegetable soup as well as salad.

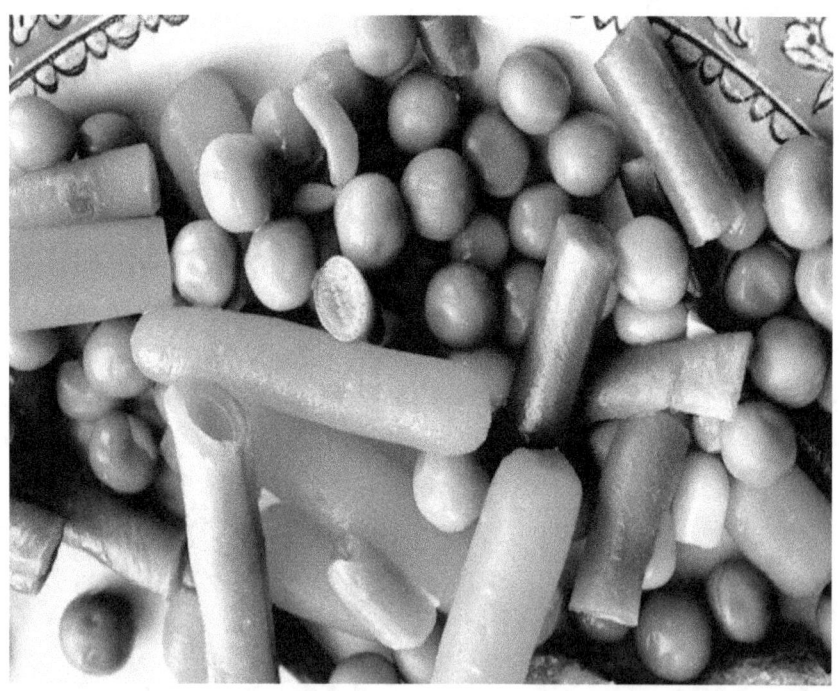

Night Treats

A glass of: Refreshing vegetable juice or a cup of herbal tea.

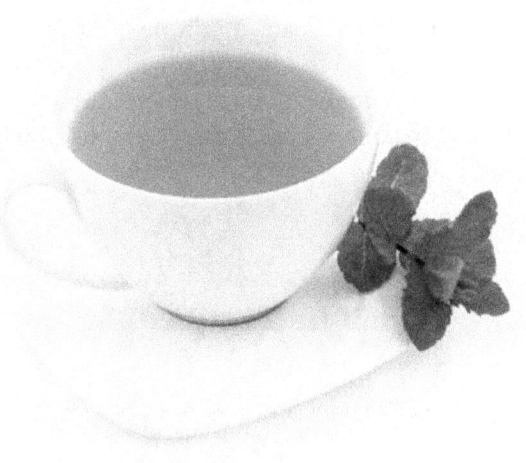

By following the steps laid out, you are helping your body to reach a smooth change from vegetable and fruit juices to lightly cooked veggies and soups as you go back to a normal and balanced diet in a safe and healthy way.

Juice fasting provides several health benefits, especially the chance for the body to relax from digestive processes. Juicing enables the body's energy to focus on purifying itself through removing toxins, waste and lifeless cells.

The minerals, vitamins as well as other nutritional elements the body gets from juice fasting are used in repairing, fixing, toning and cleaning the entire body. When breaking a juice fast, you should always do it in a way that your physical body will continue to get rid of toxins.

This is achieved by gradually breaking the fasting process as you allow your body to change from cleansing mode back to its normal digestive mode. It's necessary to follow along with your instincts as the body knows best. The human's body is clever and it will let you know whether you are breaking the juice fast the right or wrong way.

Don't Be Tempted

Moreover, don't be tempted to have foods and beverages you were craving on your fast. As your stomach is now accustomed to only having vegetable and fruit juices for quite some time, this can actually create digestive problems.

If you did a prolonged juice fast, take more preventative measures and reintroduce food into your body in a much slower way, as well as in small portions.

It is recommended that you continue your meals in small servings or even uncooked (raw) during the first few days of breaking your fast. Avoid salt, foods rich in fats and greasy foods, starch and processed sugar, as these can cause nausea and headaches or vomiting.

Instead, pick organic fresh fruits and steamed veggies. Also, try to chew your foods well as the enzymes found in your saliva will assist in the digestive process. This will cause less strain on your gastrointestinal system while it's still returning to its normal mode.

Another amazing way to break your juice fast correctly is to drink fruit and vegetable juices while gradually adding organic raw vegetables and fruits with high-water content-- like tomatoes and grapes into your daily diet.

As for your meals; you can also add raw light salads with dressing, or maybe some light vegetable soups. Increase the amount of food you eat gradually over the next two to three days.

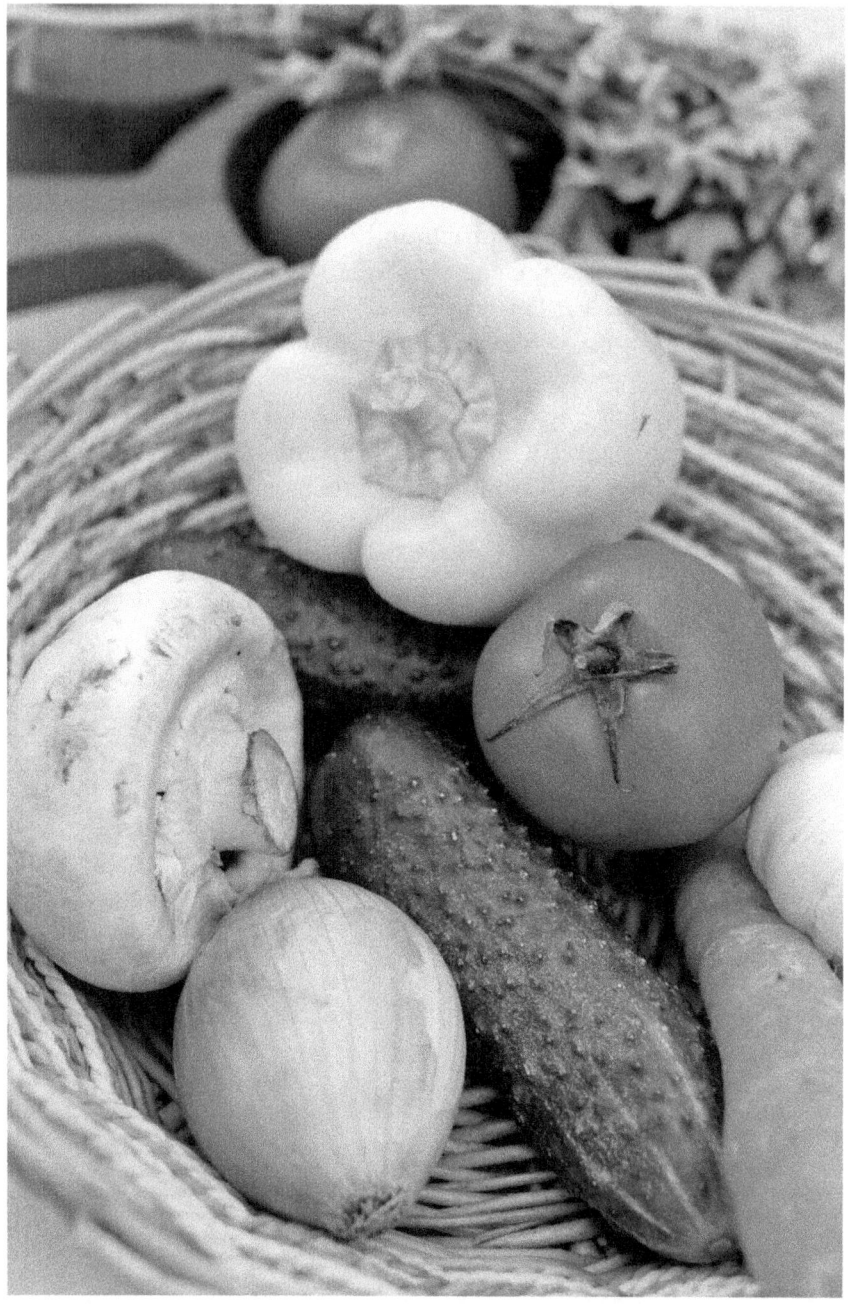

CHAPTER 19

Detox Recipes

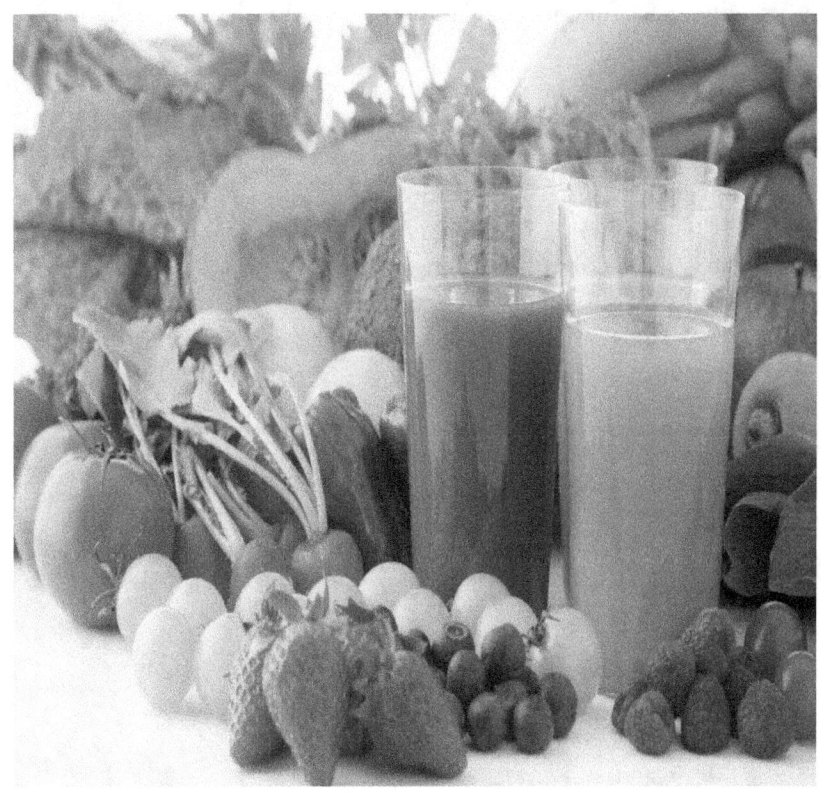

Tomato Juice Detox

Health Benefits:

Tomatoes are a natural diuretic that is full of antioxidants, and dietary fiber. Helping the metabolic process, and the gastrointestinal system, a detoxification function is stimulated by tomatoes in the liver and lungs.

Tomatoes are high in nutrition and vitamin A, vitamin C, vitamin K, and vitamin B6. Tomatoes contain many essential minerals like thiamin, folate, magnesium, niacin, phosphorus and copper.

Tomatoes also contain nutrients which help the defense mechanisms by destroying the free radicals found in the blood stream that cause damage to cells. This vegetable has also been utilized to treat heart disease. Fresh and delicious, tomato juice is excellent for an early morning pick-me up, or an afternoon snack.

Ingredients:

2 carrots
1/ 4 onion
2 celery stalks
2 tomatoes
1/ 2 of ginger

Direction:

Wash all the ingredients

Chop up the carrots, ginger, tomatoes, celery and onion into small pieces. Place all the ingredients into the juicer and blend. Drink immediately.

Nutmeg Elixir

Health Benefits:

Full of fiber and manganese, removing excess gas in the bowels, nutmeg alleviates irritable bowel syndrome and flatulence. Nutmeg juice is full of many nutrients like calcium and iron. Cleaning out the toxins in the liver, nutmeg is powerful in preventing and dissolving kidney stones.

Abundant in antibacterial properties, nutmeg is known to cleanse the bacteria in the mouth caused by halitosis or bad breath. Nutmeg is a spice that's normally used to garnish desserts and in cooked food. It's full of flavor and high in nutritional value. Nutmeg juice can be consumed throughout the day.

Ingredients:

4 apples
2 parsnips
3 teaspoons of nutmeg

Direction:

Wash all the ingredients

Cut and core the apples. Chop up the parsnips and add all the ingredients as well as the nutmeg in the juicer. Blend for one minute.

Rhubarb Juice

Health Benefits:

Rhubarb is effective in promoting internal health. In addition, rhubarb contains lots of nutritional elements such as vitamin K, vitamin C, calcium potassium, magnesium and thiamin. Rhubarb is high in vitamin C and dietary fiber.

This vegetable contains many antioxidant, anti-inflammatory and anti-allergic activities; it has also been used as a treatment for heart condition. Rhubarb juice is great for any time of the day as a snack or just to boost energy.

Ingredients:

4 large apples
7 large carrots
1 lb of cranberries
1 stalk of rhubarb

Direction:

Wash all the ingredients

Trim the ends off of the rhubarb and remove any leaves, cut and core the apples. Begin adding the ingredients to the juicer one at a time. Add ice cubes if desired and drink immediately.

Strawberry Kiwi Juice

Health Benefits:

Strawberries is used as a treatment against inflammatory illnesses, it is also used to treat asthma, degenerative joint disease and atherosclerosis. Modulating the digestive system, this fruit can lower blood pressure and prevent overeating.

Consisting several minerals and vitamins, strawberries contains manganese, Vitamin A, vitamin C, alpha and beta-carotene, potassium, and folate. Strawberries are high in dietary fiber, zinc, and antioxidants. Improving the immune system, strawberries fight infectious diseases such as a cold and flu. This juice is healthy and is best consumed in the morning.

Ingredients:

2 cups of strawberries
1 kiwi
2 apples

Direction:

Wash all of the ingredients

Cut off both ends of the kiwi. Then separate the kiwi's skin from the fruit. Now cut the apples into half and remove the core from its center. Blend all the ingredients and drink immediately.

Watercress Cleanse

Health Benefits:

Watercress flushes out impurities from the body; it is a seasonal vegetable that is full of antioxidants, protein, as well as vitamin b5. Stimulating salivary, gastric secretions and the regulation of the intestines tract.

Packed with important nutrients watercress has folic, protein, copper, riboflavin, manganese, potassium, thiamin, vitamin A, vitamin C, vitamin E, and vitamin b 6 in it.

Watercress treats and prevents chronic bronchitis and is also known to modify bronchial secretions while exerting an expectorant effect. Watercress is likewise an active remedy against degenerative and chronic diseases.

Watercress is an edible plant that is commonly found in salads. Known for its peppery and tangy flavor, this juice is a favorite among many. As a high source of vitamins, watercress is a blend that can be consumed during any time of the day.

Ingredients:

2 watercress stalks
1 stalk of broccoli
3 cups of spinach
3 oranges

Direction:

Wash all the ingredients

Cut up the broccoli florets and place them inside the juicer then cut up the spinach and watercress into small pieces to fit in the juicer. Next peel and cut the oranges into small sections. Place the ingredients in one at a time.

Guava Juice Glory

Health Benefits:

This sweet and juicy fruit is rich in fiber and vitamin C. Containing lots of astringents, guava relaxes the intestines and promotes the digestive regularity. Combating free radicals, guava helps in preventing age associated chronic diseases, such as atrophic arthritis, Alzheimer's, cardiovascular disease and cataracts.

As a rich source of nutrients, guava has iron, magnesium mineral, phosphorus, zinc, vitamin E and vitamin K, potassium, copper and calcium. Conditioning and toning the intestinal device, these nutrients aid to eliminate poisons and chemicals.

Ingredients:

1 kiwi fruit
1 guava
2 grapefruits

Direction:

Wash all the ingredients

Peel and cut the kiwi and grapefruits. Then cut up the guava and place all of the ingredients inside the juicer. Mix until the mixture is smooth.

Fruity Fennel Juice

Health Benefits:

The roughage of fennel seeds behaves as a laxative, flushing out the bowels and stimulating the movement of the intestines, thus helping proper excretion. Fennel additionally shields the eyes from illnesses and inflammation associated with aging.

Consisting lots of wholesome nutrients like iron, niacin, phosphorus, copper and magnesium. Fennel has carminative properties of aspartic acid that may treat flatulence and eliminate gasses of the stomach. Fennel is an herbaceous plant that is widely used in cooking.

This herbaceous plant makes one of the tastiest juices and is well-known for its distinctive and strong flavor. Packaged with lots of minerals and vitamins, fennel juice is very good for practically any time of the day.

Ingredients:

2 medium fennel bulbs
2 Comice pears

Direction:

Wash all the ingredients

Cut and core the Comice pears and then, chop up the fennel bulbs and begin placing all of the ingredients into the juicer. As soon as it's finished, mix well.

Broccoli Sunrise

Health Benefits:

Broccoli flushes out toxins in the gastrointestinal system helping in the regulation of bowel movements. Broccoli is also a super vegetable which is full of anti-oxidants, fiber and lutein. Lutein is an anti-oxidant that is practically the same as beta carotene.

Consisting many vital nutritional elements and vitamins, broccoli is an excellent source of calcium, niacin, thiamin, riboflavin, iron, zinc, vitamin A and vitamin B 6. Broccoli is effective in fighting against vision disorders; it is also used to treat cataracts.

Broccoli is also a good source of vitamin in the treatment of cancer. Broccoli is a popular vegetable that is commonly eaten as a side dish. Surprisingly delicious, this juice has a bold and savory taste. This juice can be consumed any time of the day but is best in the morning.

Ingredients:

1 broccoli stalk
3 celery stalks
1 green orange

Direction:

Wash all the ingredients

Peel and cut the orange. Begin placing the ingredients in one at a time. Blend until smooth and drink immediately.

Lime Detox

Health Benefits:

Lime is full of citric acid. Stimulating the gastrointestinal system and increasing the secretion of digestive juices, like acids and bile, limes additionally promote peristaltic activity.

Lime juice is also high in several nutrients like potassium, calcium, iron, vitamin C and vitamin A. This fruit include several anti-oxidants, anti-biotic and disinfectant abilities; they additionally have been used for skincare including rashes clearing out the excretory system, the acids found in lime wash and clear off the tracts.

Limes are a fruit that is commonly eaten raw, in salads, or squeezed to add flavor to specific foods. Known for the sharp flavor, limes has several health benefits and can be consumed throughout the day.

Ingredients:

8 tablespoons of honey
4 white grapes
1 liter water
1 lime

Direction:

Wash all the ingredients

Peel and cut the lime into 4 small pieces. Place all the ingredients into the juicer and mix until the mixture is smooth. Add ice cubes if needed.

Asparagus Juice Detox

Health Benefits:

Asparagus is full of polypeptides, fiber and antioxidants. Asparagus helps the body gets rid of waste effectively and rapidly, while repairing skin disorders, vision issues as well as the nervous system.

As a natural diuretic, this vegetable flushes out toxins from the body encouraging maximum kidney health. Asparagus includes several antioxidants which make it beneficial in remedies to reduce tumors and prevent cancer. Asparagus as several essential vitamins and minerals such as folic acid, calcium, vitamin C, niacin, copper and iron.

Abundant and strong, asparagus juice is among the most delicious drinks accessible to date. Asparagus has several essential minerals and vitamins and is best with other sweet fruits. This vegetable is one of the best for detoxing.

Ingredients:

1 lemon
9 stalks of asparagus
1 tsp olive oil

Direction:

Wash all ingredients

Remove the skin from the lemon; now place the asparagus, olive oil and lemon into the juicer. Blend until the juices texture is smooth. Add ice cubes if desired and drink immediately.

Apple And Cucumber Detox

Health Benefits:

The health benefits of Cucumber are primarily located in its skin, which includes potassium, silica, folic acid, magnesium, molybdenum, vitamins A and vitamins C. Containing high alkaline levels, cucumbers regulate the physical body's blood pH and reduces the effects of acidity level.

Cucumber juice is a diuretic that is full of protein, fiber, and calcium. Contributing to the regulation of the human body and blood pressure, cucumbers also eliminate toxins from the body. This delicious vegetable has been used for diabetic patients.

Ingredients:

1 cucumber
4 apples
8 carrots
ginger root   (a small piece)

Direction:

Wash all the ingredients

Cut the ginger root into half pieces, remove the apple core and then cut up the apples and cucumbers into four pieces. Begin juicing the ingredients one piece at a time; apple piece first then the carrots, add the ginger last. Add ice if desired and drink immediately.

Ginger Root Delight

Health Benefits:

Ginger root consist of several vitamins and minerals such as copper, manganese, iron, potassium, magnesium, phosphorus, sodium, zinc, selenium, vitamin E, vitamin C and vitamin K. Consists of anti-inflammatory properties, ginger has more than twelve kinds of antioxidants, which makes it an excellent treatment for different kinds of illnesses.

Ginger root has also been used to treat rheumatic and inflammatory illnesses. Ginger is a diuretic that's full of antioxidants, protein and calcium. A great cure for nausea, and stomach upset, ginger is good for inducing blood circulation throughout the body.

Ingredients:

2 oranges

1 pineapple

ginger root   (a small piece)

Direction:

Wash all the ingredients

Remove the crown and base from pineapple and carefully cut the rind off the pineapple. Next, chop the pineapple into chunky pieces and set aside.

Peel the skin from the oranges and slice into small sections to fit into the juicer. Now cut up the ginger root into smaller pieces and place all the ingredients into the juicer. Begin juicing. Drink immediately.

Celery Juice Detox

Health Benefits:

Celery is a natural cleanser abundant in iron, vitamin C and folic acid. Celery contains lots of dietary properties such as calcium, magnesium, phosphorus, vitamin A, thiamin and vitamin B2.

Accentuating the activity of white blood cells, celery includes coumarin which is a class of antioxidants that have been used to fight cancer. Additionally Celery juice also assists in breaking the removal of urinary and gall-bladder stones. Actively modulating the gastrointestinal system, Celery softens stools and induces a normality of bowel movements.

Ingredients:

1 apple

2 stalks of celery

1/ 2 broccoli stalk

5 carrots

Direction:

Wash all the ingredients

Cut the celery, carrots and broccoli into pieces, then slice and core the apple. Begin juicing all the ingredients. Drink immediately.

Kale Morning Glory

Health Benefits:

Kale is a natural source for phytonutrient lutein and also antioxidant carotenoid. Kale is a very powerful vegetable that flushes out toxins in the body by stimulating the liver detox enzymes. Kale can be used in the treatment against cancer, due to the high-content of anti-oxidants.

It is a leafy vegetable that is full of omega-3 and antioxidants. Kale is consists of phytochemicals that regulate the immune system. Including several essential vitamins and minerals, kale is an excellent way to obtain iron, potassium, vitamins A, vitamin C, vitamin K, calcium, manganese and copper.

Ingredients:

2 cups of kale

1 grapefruit

2 green apples

1 cup of blueberries

4 stalks of celery

Direction:

Wash all the ingredients

Cut and core the apples, kale and celery. Peel the grapefruit and cut in small pieces to fit easily into the juicer. Process all the ingredients in the juicer.

Sweet Morning Mango Juice

Mangos are a sweet fleshy fruit which is high in beta-carotene and antioxidants, and dietary fiber. As a natural diuretic, mangos flush out toxins in the human body, cleansing both digestive system and the urinary tract. It is an excellent source of iron, zinc and phosphorus, vitamin A, vitamin C, folate, calcium, and copper.

Displaying high antibacterial action, mangos possess anti-inflammatory and tonic attributes that assist in fixing many viral ailments. Naturally healthy, mangos are a great source of many essential minerals and vitamins.

Mangos are a favorite among many individuals, it is very popular because of its sweet taste and soft feel; it can be used in fruit salad or eaten raw. Drink mango juice only in the morning or afternoon.

Ingredients:

1 mango   (small or medium size)

1 orange

1 banana

2 kiwis

Direction:

Wash all the ingredients

Peel the mango, orange, banana, kiwi, and then cut them into pieces. Place all the ingredients in the juicer.

Watermelon Juice Cleanse

Health Benefits:

There are lots of healthful properties associated with watermelons as they've vitamin A, vitamin C and potassium. Used in treating bladder infections, also to detox the body, water melons are among the very best fruits to use in a detox.

Watermelon is a diuretic that's high in antioxidants, fiber and lycopene. The anti-oxidants in watermelons lower the potential risk of rheumatoid arthritis, heart disease and colon cancer. Watermelon gives you lots of energy! It is best consumed in the morning.

Ingredients:

1 apple

1/ 8 large watermelon

8 strawberries

Direction:

Wash all the ingredients

Remove the outer skin from the watermelon. Cut the watermelon into small. Now cut the apple and remove its core. Begin juicing and drink immediately.

Cucumber And Carrot Juice

Health Benefits:

Carrots are rich in beta carotene, antioxidants and dietary fiber. Made up of different minerals, this vegetable is saturated in potassium, copper, manganese, calcium and phosphorous. Good for eye health, bone development and reproduction, one carrot provides more than the daily dietary requirement for vitamin A.

Carrots also generate white blood cells that help control the immune system by destroying microorganisms (bacteria) that cause medical conditions and infections. Carrot juice can be consumed throughout the day; it is one of the most delicious juices filled with lots of vitamins and minerals.

Ingredients:

8 large carrots

2 large cucumbers

lemon wedge   (1/ 2)

Direction:

Wash all the ingredients

Place the cucumber, carrot and peeled lemon inside the juicer. Press start on your juicer and enjoy.

Cabbage Juice

Health Benefits:

Cabbage is high in vitamin C and dietary fiber. This leafy vegetable includes extremely high levels of fiber which helps retain water and terrific for the intestinal system. Therefore, it is effective in treating constipation and other health issues.

Rich in iodine, cabbage boosts brain function as well as the nervous system, and keeps the endocrine glands in proper condition. Consisting of several nutritional benefits, cabbage contains polypeptides, thiamin, phosphorus, copper, vitamin A, vitamin b 6, folic acid and magnesium. High in sulphur, cabbage is very effective in fighting against illnesses.

Cabbage is a leafy vegetable that's mainly eaten in salads. Known for its crunchy and rich taste, cabbage juice is a popular mixture among lots of people. High in vitamins and minerals cabbage juice can be consumed throughout the day.

Ingredients:

1/ 2 of cabbage

5 almonds

3 oranges

Direction:

Wash all the ingredients

Slice the cabbage into 4 quarters, peel and cut the orange into small pieces to easily fit into the juicer. Then add the almonds and all the other ingredients to the juicer. Mix until the mixture is smooth.

Blueberry And Cantaloupe Juice

Health Benefits:

Blueberries contain several nutritional elements such as calcium, iron, manganese, vitamin A, vitamin C, vitamin E, vitamin K, vitamin B6, phosphorus and copper. Blueberries additionally contain anthocyanin, an anti-oxidant plant pigment that contributes to its distinguishing color.

It is also a diuretic that is full of dietary fiber, antioxidants, and tannins. Eliminating bacteria and viruses, blueberries prevent bladder infections and detox the body. This fruit has also been used to combat diabetes and urinary tract infection. Blueberries are packed with many vitamins and minerals, this juice can be consumed throughout the day.

Ingredients:

1/ 2 cantaloupe

1 cup of blueberries

3 apples

Direction:

Wash all the ingredients

Peel the apple and remove the core and then cut the netted skin off of the cantaloupe. Place all the ingredients into the juicer. Add ice cubes if desired and drink immediately.

Sweet Radish Juice

Health Benefits:

Radishes are reddish vegetables that are high in vitamin C and dietary fiber. Radishes help in digestion stimulating the production of bile, liver and gallbladder health. Radishes also contain many important nutrients like calcium, vitamin A, vitamin B, and vitamin K, iron, copper, potassium, phosphorus and zinc.

Radishes purify the blood and increase oxygen levels. Many researchers have stated that antioxidants reduce cholesterol levels in the body which lowers the danger of heart issues. Radishes are root vegetables that can be eaten uncooked/raw. With its strong and sweet flavor this juice can be consumed throughout the day to boots your energy level.

Ingredients:

1 beet

1 carrot

1 cabbage leaf

1 radish

1 apple

Direction:

Wash all the ingredients

Remove all the skin from the beet and then chop it into small chunky pieces, cut off the leaves, stem, and roots of the radish. Now, cut open the apple and remove the core. Chop up the cabbage leaves and place all the ingredients in the juicer.

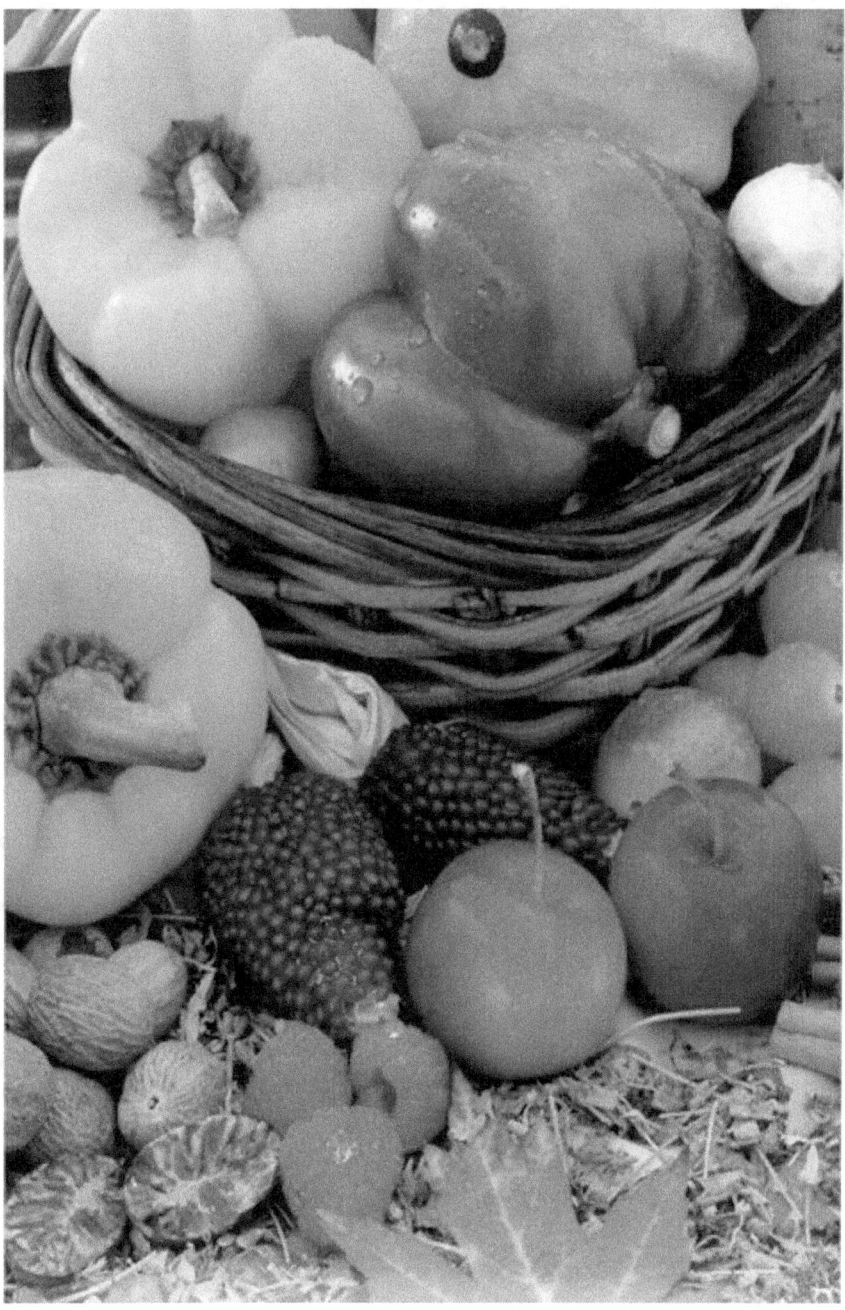

CHAPTER 20

Weight Loss Juicing Recipes

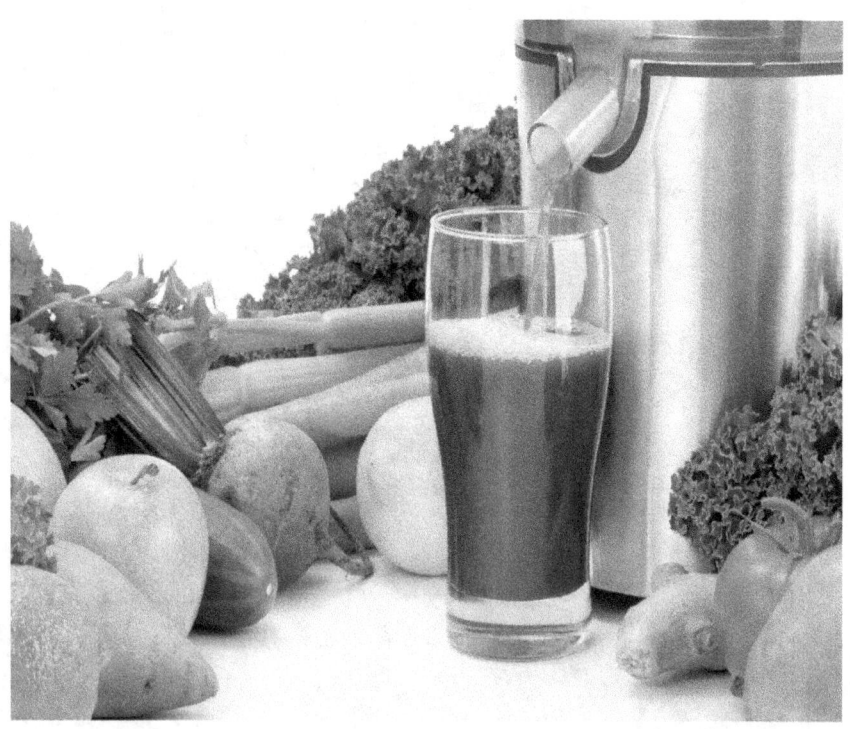

BEFORE YOU START

A juice fast is one of the best approaches to start a weight loss plan. It'll flush the toxins from your body and prepare it to process the healthy foods that you're going to be putting in it. A clean system likewise has lots of energy and is easier to use the oxygen that it gets during exercise.

Don't think of the juice fast as a diet or just a weight loss plan. The weight loss that you'll experience from juicing and then eating healthful foods and physical exercise on a normal basis is just another side effect of a body that's working properly.

You owe it to yourself; your health and well-being as well as your appearances. You'll feel and see the difference in your body and will want to stick with it more if you think of it that way instead of as a short-cut to a smaller size dress.

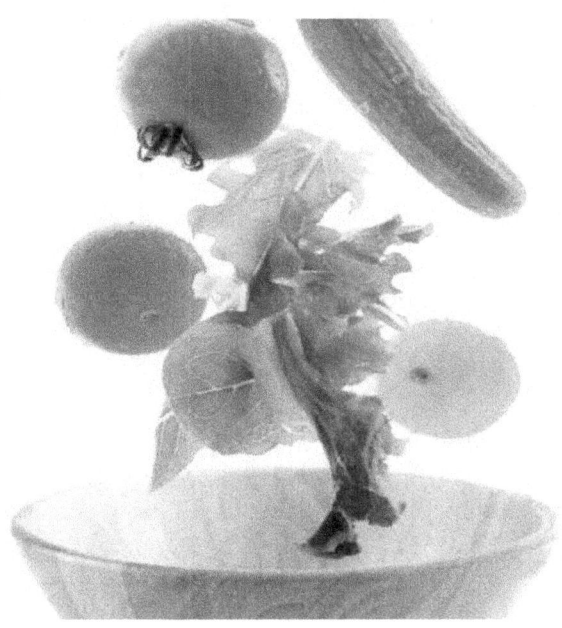

Energy Rush

Blood sugar levels drop when the muscles and liver breakdown of glycogen stores into glucose, releasing it into the tissues. This can lead to fatigue as well as depression, so it is vital that you maintain your blood sugar levels to be able to function consistently.

Fruits contain high amounts of natural sugar therefore try to include vegetable juices as well. Cinnamon is known, for stabilizing blood sugar. To add an extra boost of glucose- regulating chromium, stir 1 teaspoon of raw wheat germ into the finished juice.

Ingredients:

4 cups spinach
2 apples
1 yellow pepper
1 teaspoon cinnamon

Direction:

Wash all the ingredients

Core the apples and pepper and slice in half. Now add all the ingredients in the juicer including the cinnamon. Serve in a tall glass. If desired add ice cubes.

Parsnip Juice

Health Benefits:

Parsnips are high in dietary fiber and protein. As a natural diuretic, parsnips helps with nerve function and regulate blood pressure. This vegetable has many essential vitamins and minerals such as vitamin C and vitamin K, folic acid, manganese, potassium. With several antibacterial properties, parsnips reduce inflammation in the body. Parsnips juice is best in the afternoon or evening.

Ingredients:

1 teaspoon of nutmeg
2 Parsnips
4 Apples

Direction:

Wash all the ingredients

Cut the apples, parsnips and the nutmeg. Add all the ingredients inside the juicer. Blend until smooth and drink immediately.

Iron Boost

Folic acid builds up red blood cells, chlorophyll helps to combat fatigue, spirulina provides a valuable boost of vitamins B12.

Ingredients

3 cups spinach
2 cups of parsley
2 carrots
1 teaspoon of spirulina

Directions

Wash all the ingredients

Juice the spinach, parsley and carrots and stir in the spirulina. Serve in a tall glass and drink immediately.

Celery Burst Juice

Ingredients:

2 apples
4 celery stalks
2 limes

Direction:

Wash all the ingredients

Add the celery, apples and limes to the juicer. Stir and drink immediately.

Grapefruit Punch Juice

Ingredients:

1 grapefruit
1 orange
1 lemon

Direction:

Wash all the ingredients

Add the grapefruit, orange and lemon to the juicer. Add ice cubes and stir well.

Vitality Boost Juice

The cayenne pepper will help boost the metabolism to give you energy throughout the day.

Ingredients:

2 celery stalks
½ lemon
¼ teaspoon cayenne pepper
1 teaspoon grated horseradish
½ lime

Direction:

Wash all the ingredients

Add the tomatoes, celery, lime, lemon, cayenne pepper and horseradish in the juicer. Blend and drink immediately.

On The Go

Health Benefits:

Plums are high in antioxidants and dietary fiber. Assisting in the absorption and production of iron in the body, plums maintain proper blood flow throughout the body. Plums also contains many vital nutrients, they are full of beta carotene, niacin, vitamin A, vitamin C, thiamin and potassium. Plums can be consumed throughout the day.

Ingredients:

4 apples
6 plums
1 mango

Direction:

Wash all the ingredients

Cut the mango, apples and the plums and slice into small chunks. Add all the ingredients into the juicer. Add ice cubes and serve in a tall glass.

Metabolism Boost Juice

Ingredients:

½ lemon
½-inch ginger
½ cup cranberries
½ sweet potato
1 handful wheatgrass

Direction:

Wash all the ingredients

Add all the ingredients to the juicer. Blend until smooth then pour into a glass, stir well and enjoy.

Jalapeno Spice Juice

Ingredients:

½ jalapeno pepper
2 tomatoes
1 lemon
3 celery stalks
2 carrots

Direction:

Wash all the ingredients

Peel the lemon and chop the celery, carrots, and tomatoes. Now add all the ingredients into the juicer including the jalapeno. Begin to blend all the ingredients. Stir well and enjoy.

Green Rocket

Ingredients:

½ teaspoon cayenne pepper
1 cucumber
3 lemons
1 cup water

Direction:

Wash all the ingredients

Peel the lemon and the cucumber. Blend the lemon and cucumber in the juicer. Now add the water and cayenne pepper to the juice. Stir well and drink immediately.

Bumpy Ride

Ingredients:

1 apple
1 celery stalk
½ cucumber
½-inch piece ginger
¼ cup kale leaves
¼ head lettuce
¼ fennel bulb
¼ lemon
¼ cup spinach

Direction:

Wash all the ingredients

Peel the ginger, lemon and cucumber. Remove the core from the apple. Now begin to add the ingredients into the juicer one at a time. Stir well and serve in a tall glass with ice cubes.

Cool Ginger

Ingredients:

2 pears
1 cucumber
½-inch piece ginger
1 apple

Direction:

Wash all the ingredients

Peel the skin from the ginger, cucumber and peer. Now remove the core from the pear and apple. Begin to add all the ingredients into the juicer one at a time. Stir well and serve in a tall glass with ice cubes.

Pineapple Flush

Health Benefits:

Having lots of dietary benefits such as thiamine, manganese, manganese, copper, potassium, vitamin B6, and vitamin C. Good for fighting cold and flu, pineapples have natural healing properties that suppress coughs and breakdown mucus.

Pineapples are high in dietary fiber, and calcium. Helping with food digestion, the bromelain found in pineapples lessen bloating, irritable bowel syndrome, gas, constipation, and nausea. Packed with many nutritional benefits, this juice can be consumed in the morning or afternoon.

Ingredients:

1/ 2 of pineapple
2 bananas
3 oranges

Direction:

Wash all the ingredients

Cut off the top and bottom of the pineapple. Remove the rind and cut in halves. Peel and slice the banana and orange in small chunks. Add all the ingredients into the juicer. Add ice cubes and drink immediately.

Easy Lettuce Juice

Health Benefits:

Packed with lots of essential vitamins and minerals, lettuce is abundant in dietary fiber and potassium. The levels of antioxidants this juice has contributed to digestive health promoting regularity in the human body.

Moreover, Lettuce also has plenty of nutrients found in vitamin C, vitamin E, vitamin K, copper, manganese, iron, potassium, folic acid, and phosphorus. Additionally, lettuce helps when performing aerobics exercise and lowers hypertension significantly.

Ingredients:

2 oranges
6 romaine lettuce leaves

Direction:

Wash all the ingredients

Peel the oranges and cut into halve. Chop up the lettuce leaves. Now begin to place all of the ingredients into the juicer. Blend until smooth. Serve into a tall glass and enjoy.

Garlic Glory

Ingredients:

2 green onions
2 garlic cloves
3 oregano leaves
4 basil leaves
2 tomatoes
1 green bell pepper

Direction:

Wash all the ingredients

Add the garlic, tomatoes, basil, bell pepper, green onions and oregano in the juicer. Now begin to blend all the ingredients. Enjoy

Moody Blues

Health Benefits:

Known for Killing bacteria and viruses, blackberries prevent bladder infections and flush out poisonous toxins from the body. Blackberries are high in dietary tannic acids, fiber, and antioxidants. This fruit have several nutritional elements such as copper, manganese, iron, phosphorus and calcium, vitamin E, vitamin A, vitamin C, vitamin K, and vitamin b-6.

Additionally, blackberries also contain anthocyanin, an antioxidant plant pigment that that contributes to its unique color. This fruit in addition has been used to fight diabetes, urinary tract infection, and aging. Blackberries are good sources of folic acid. Full with lots of vitamins and minerals, this juice can be consumed any time of the day.

Ingredients:

1 orange
4 cups of blackberries
1 apple
4 tbsp. of honey

Direction:

Wash all the ingredients

Remove the core from the apple and peel the orange. Next cut them into chunky portions and begin placing all the ingredients into the juicer. Mix well and serve into a tall glass and enjoy.

Cool Down Juice

Health Benefits:

Papayas consist of many essential vitamins and minerals like iron, vitamin B6, folate, potassium, and thiamin. Additionally, papayas have been utilized to lessen cholesterol. Papayas are rich in anti-oxidants, calcium, and fiber.

As a natural diuretic, they have been great for the gastrointestinal system and for alleviating constipation. Sparking the production of white blood cells, papayas assist the immune system and prevent diseases. Packed with several vitamins and minerals this juice is best consumed throughout the day as it boosts the immune system and gives you lots of energy.

Ingredients:

1 orange
2 papayas
1 pineapple

Direction:

Wash all the ingredients

Remove all the skin from the papaya and discard any seeds with a teaspoon. Next peel the orange and the pineapple. Now remove the rind from the pineapple. Cut the pineapple, orange and papaya in small portions. Now begin to place all the ingredients into the juicer one at a time. Mix well and serve into a tall glass and enjoy.

Sleep Tight

Health Benefits:

Grapes are full of zinc, antioxidants and dietary fiber. Regulating the digestive system, these fruits can reduce blood pressure and stop overeating. Comprising many vitamins and minerals, grapes provide Vitamin A, vitamin C, alpha and beta carotene, folate, potassium, and manganese. Grapes act as a cure against inflammatory illnesses, to handle atherosclerosis, osteoarthritis and asthma. Grapes give a boost of blood sugar, which can help to induce sleep. This juice is healthy and is best consumed in the morning or afternoon.

Ingredients:

2 cups of grapes
3 Pears
24 baby carrots

Direction:

Wash all the ingredients

Cut and core the pears. Begin placing all of the ingredients into the juicer. Mix well and serve in a tall glass.

Celtuce Juice

Health Benefits:

Celtuce is a vegetable that's abundant in vitamin C, folic acid and iron. Celtuce regulates the gastrointestinal system by regulating bowel movements and softens stools. Celtuce also contains many dietary properties like phosphorus, magnesium, vitamin B 2, vitamin A, calcium and thiamin.

This vegetable improves white blood cells and also contains coumarins which are a course of antioxidants that have been used to fight cancer. Celtuce juice can be consumed any time of the day.

Ingredients:

1 bunch of celtuce leaves
1 large green cabbage
2 pears
1 ginger root

Direction:

Wash all the ingredients

Cut and core the pears. Chop the cabbage and the celtuce leaves. Remove the skin from the ginger root. Place all of the ingredients into the juicer and blend until smooth. Serve in a tall glass and drink immediately.

Loosen Up Chili Juice

Health Benefits:

Chili peppers consist of many essential nutrients such as potassium, magnesium, vitamin E, vitamin A, vitamin C, vitamin K, vitamin b 6, manganese, niacin and riboflavin.

Moreover, chili peppers contain capsaicin which assists the immune system having its antibacterial, anti-carcinogenic, analgesic and antidiuretic properties. Boosting the metabolic process, chili peppers trigger the entire body to burn off calories quickly. This juice is fantastic! And can be consumed any time of the day.

Ingredients:

2 chili peppers
1 teaspoon of ginger
2 cups of spinach
2 celery stalks
3 carrots
1/ 2 lime

Direction:

Wash all the ingredients

Remove the skin from the ginger, peel the lime and cut it in half. Now chop up the peppers, spinach leaves and celery stalks. Begin adding all the ingredients to the juicer. Blend until smooth. Serve in a glass and drink immediately.

Cantaloupe Juice

Health Benefits:

Cantaloupes are high in dietary fiber, beta carotene and anti-oxidants. As a natural diuretic, cantaloupes aids in cleansing the body, stimulating white blood cells; this fruit helps the immune system by destroying viruses and bacteria.

While delivering several nutrients to the body cantaloupes contains niacin, potassium, vitamin A, vitamin B, vitamin C, and folic acid. Cantaloupe is known for its lightly sweet taste and juicy texture. Delivering many nutritional benefits, this drink is best in the morning, and the afternoon as it delivers high energy and vitality.

Ingredients:

1/ 2 cantaloupe
2 carrots
1 banana

Direction:

Wash all the ingredients

Remove the rind off the cantaloupe. Peel the banana. Now chop the banana and cantaloupe into chunks. Now begin to place all the ingredients into the juicer. Serve in a tall glass and drink immediately.

Flat Abs

Health Benefits:

Consisting lots of health properties such as potassium, magnesium, vitamin A, vitamin C, vitamin E, and vitamin B, calcium, manganese, zinc and iron dandelion leaves are high in anti-oxidants and protein. As a natural diuretic, dandelion leaves remove toxins from the kidneys and also the urinary system.

Dandelion helps to increase the absorption of magnesium and calcium in the body. In addition, these green leaves assist the digestive system by improving the growth of healthy bacteria in the body. Dandelion leaves can be consumed any time of day.

Ingredients:

3 cups of dandelion leaves
1 cup of spinach
1 carrot
1 cucumber
1 pear

Direction:

Wash all the ingredients

Cut the pear and remove the core, then remove the skin from the cucumber. Now add all the ingredients into the juicer. Mix well and drink immediately.

Tangy Zucchini Juice

Health Benefits:

Made up of several minerals, Zucchini is saturated in protein, vitamin C, vitamin K, vitamin b 6, thiamin, niacin, copper and folic acid. Moreover, this fresh vegetable also generate white blood cells that assist modulate the immune system by destroying bacteria that cause sicknesses and disease.

Zucchini is abundant in nutritional fiber and anti-oxidants. Consisting of natural inflammatory properties, Zucchini also helps prevent asthma and bruising in the body. Packed with many vitamins and minerals, Zucchini Juice can be consumed anytime of the day.

Ingredients:

1 tbsp. of honey
1 cup of zucchini
1 cup butternut squash

Direction:

Wash all the ingredients

Remove the skin from the zucchini and butternut squash and chop into small chunks. Begin to put all the ingredients into the juicer one at a time. Blend until smooth and drink immediately.

Refreshing Beet juice

Health Benefits:

Beet juice is a dark purplish red juice produced from beetroot. Packed with lots of essential vitamins and minerals, this juice is ideal when mixed with sweet fruits. Beet juice contributes to cardiovascular health as well as the stimulation of red blood cells.

Moreover, beetroot likewise help lowers high blood pressure and aid in the advancement of athletic performance. Beets are abundant in fiber, antioxidants and high complex carbohydrates.

Ingredients:

1 apple
2 carrots
1/ 2 beet

Direction:

Wash all the ingredients

Remove the apple core; peel the beets, and apples. Now place all of the ingredients into the juicer one at a time. Blend until smooth. Add ice cubes and drink immediately.

Sweet And Sour Mix

Health Benefits:

Pears are high in dietary fiber and protein. While the glucose and sugar provide plenty of energy to the human body, bowel movements are regulated by natural diuretic pectin.

Delivering a high source of nutrients, pears contain vitamin C, vitamin A, vitamin K, calcium and potassium. Pears have antioxidant, ant-carcinogen and glutathione which can prevent hypertension or a stroke. Pear juice can be consumed any time of day.

Ingredients:

1 pear
1 celery stalk
1 kiwi
6 oz. of water
1/ 2 of grapefruit
1 tbsp. of honey
1 tbsp. of oatmeal

Direction:

Wash all the ingredients

Peel and cut the grapefruit, pear, kiwi and chop in chunks. Add all the ingredients including the oatmeal, water and honey into the juicer. Add ice cubes and serve in a tall glass.

Sweet And Sour Blues

Health Benefits:

An all-natural diuretic, grapefruits effectively breaks down fat and grease in the stomach, then flushes it out of the urinary and gastrointestinal systems. Grapefruits are full of antioxidants, dietary fiber and beta carotene.

Eating grapefruit on a regular base is a great way to obtain vitamin A, vitamin C, calcium potassium and iron. In addition, grapefruits are effective in reducing the acid development in the body.

Known for its exceptional flavor, grapefruits are bitter, sweet and tangy all at the same time. With several nutritional benefits this is wonderful in the early morning or afternoon; grapefruits provide enough energy to last the entire day.

Ingredients:

2 medium apples
1 medium beet
3 carrots
1 pink grapefruit

Direction:

Wash all the ingredients

Peel and cut the grapefruit. Chop the apples, carrots and beets in small chunks. Now place all of the ingredients inside the juicer. Serve into a tall glass and drink immediately.

The Lemon Mix

Health Benefits:

As a natural diuretic, lemons are full of protein, dietary fiber and citric acid. Lemon juice efficiently breaks down fatty tissue in the gut, and then flushes it out of the urinary and digestive systems. Used to reduce blood pressure and cholesterol levels, lemons neutralize free radicals in the human body preventing several types of cancer.

Lemons are extremely nutritious and contain magnesium, iron, potassium, vitamin b5, vitamin A, vitamin C, vitamin b 6 and thiamin. Having powerful antioxidants called limonoids, this fruit improve and strengthen the immune system. Packed with many essential nutrients lemon juice can be consumed any time of the day.

Ingredients:

1 lemon
1 tsp of ground ginger
9 tangerines

Direction:

Wash all the ingredients

Peel and cut the tangerines and the lemon. Now add all the ingredients into the juicer. Add ice cubes and serve in a tall glass. Drink immediately.

Vegetable Blues

Health Benefits:

Artichokes are naturally full of dietary fiber and antioxidants. As this vegetable helps in gall-bladder function, liver function and digestive function, it is an all-natural diuretic.

Artichokes also contain several vital nutrients such as niacin, folates, riboflavin, calcium, potassium, thiamin, vitamin A, vitamin C, vitamin E and vitamin K. With the ability to restore tissue, artichokes have been used to treat liver conditions. Artichokes juice can be consumed in the afternoon or evening.

Ingredients:

6 carrots
12 brussels sprouts
1/ 2 lemon
6 Jerusalem artichokes
3 cups of green beans

Direction:

Wash all the ingredients

Cut off the artichoke's stem, then chop up the artichokes, green beans and carrots. Now pull off the dry leaves and put into the juicer. Peel the lemon and cut into half. Now start adding all of the ingredients to the juicer. Blend until smooth. Drink immediately.

Easy Going

Health Benefits:

Mint is an herbaceous plant which is full of bioflavonoids, and volatile oils. Easing digestion, the saliva glands are activated by the smell of mint in the mouth, which then secretes digestive enzymes. Moreover, the mint is abundant in several nutrients such as calcium, magnesium, beta carotene, iron, vitamin A and vitamin C.

With all the natural ability to clear-up congestion, mint is utilized as a treatment for respiratory illnesses like asthma and bronchitis. Mint additionally contains enzymes which have demonstrated to aid with cancer treatments. Mint juice can be consumed in the afternoon or evening.

Ingredients:

1/ 2 slice melon
4 tablespoons of fresh mint
1 apple
3 pears

Direction:

Wash all the ingredients

Cut the melon into halves. Scoop out the seeds from the melon using a teaspoon. Cut the melon into small cubes to fit into the juicer. Remove the core from the apples and pears, slice in half and remove the stems. Now add all the ingredients into a juicer. Add ice cubes and serve in a tall glass.

Afternoon Glory

Health Benefits:

Garlic is an herb that is saturated in vitamin C and calcium. Increasing the production of in bile, garlic helps to reduce the fat deposits levels in the liver. Moreover, this juice delivers lots of nutrients to the body such as vitamin b-6, manganese, selenium and phosphorus.

Fortifying the body's defense system against allergic reactions, garlic loosens oral plaque buildup from the canal walls, and regulates blood sugar levels. Drink garlic juice in the afternoon or evening

Ingredients:

2 beets
1 clove of garlic
6 carrots
6 cups of watercress
2 red onions

Direction:

Wash all the ingredients

Remove the skin from the onions, beets and garlic and cut into chunks. Chop up the watercress. Now place all of the ingredients into the juicer. Serve in a tall glass and drink immediately.

Refreshing Eggplant Juice

Health Benefits:

Contributing to the regulation of the human body, and blood pressure, eggplant removes toxins and waste from the body. Eggplant juice is full of protein, fiber, and calcium.

The benefits of consuming eggplant are mainly located on its skin, which consist of magnesium, silica, vitamins A, C, folate, molybdenum and potassium. It is an effective treatment used for diabetes, consisting of high levels of alkaline; it controls the body's blood pH and neutralizes acidity. Eggplant produces hormone needed by beta cells during the insulin production.

Ingredients:

2 oranges
1 eggplant

Direction:

Wash all the ingredients

Cut the stem off the eggplant, peel the orange and cut into small portions. Now add all the ingredients to the juicer. Add ice cubes and serve in a tall glass. Drink immediately.

From The Author To The Reader

Make Your Own Personal Juice

Juices that is bought in the store is pasteurized, this means that all the valuable enzymes which will make your fast effective have been ruined. Likewise, additives and preservatives that are regularly used to extend the shelf-life of the juice are precisely what you're trying to flush from your system.

Organic Produce

One of the benefits of making your personal juice is that you are in control of the ingredients. Since you're fasting to get rid of poisonous toxins and waste from your body, you want to stay away from chemicals and pesticides. If you do not utilize organic produce, peeling your produce before you juice it is advised.

Drink Your Juice Immediately After Juicing

Many of the live enzymes in your juice start to die as soon as you remove the skin off the produce. It is recommended to drink your juice immediately after juicing to get the complete benefits from the produce.

Fast from Three to Five Days

An effective fast is from three to five days. There are individuals who said they did a juice cleanse for one day, however, if you want to see good results I suggest starting small; which is a three to five days cleanse, stop for a couple of days then fast for seven days, break for a couple of days, then fast for ten days.

Doing this, gives your body time to adjust and become stronger. Fasting for one day is a great way to get nutrients, but it is not ideal if you're trying to rid your system of waste and toxins. It takes about two days to empty your body of solid waste, and your body can't really start cleansing and repairing itself until that happens.

Some individuals choose to fast for weeks or even months, but this isn't recommended by most nutritionists or healthcare professionals, especially if this is your first juice fast. After seven days, your muscles begin to break down because you need protein in order to build and maintain lean muscle mass. Therefore, the ideal time frame for a juice fast without harming your body would be three to five days.

Conclusion

Along with a well-balanced diet, regular exercise, and a good attitude, the juices of greens, sprouts, fresh veggies, wheat grass and fruits can play a significant part in attaining and maintaining good health. These foods have the power to protect us from all kinds of illness by strengthening our immune systems.

Fresh fruits and vegetables stimulate our overall metabolism, keep us balanced inside and clean, and mobilize our body's defenses against many modern day environmental strains that have been proven to cause degenerative even disease.

In this modern age, biological mechanisms like the human body cannot strive, or even survive, on synthetic processed foods and chemicals. Observing the pale complexions, lethargic activities, and unhealthiness of people who eat this way, one can simply imagine the long-term effect this type of diet will have on the world's population-if left unattended.

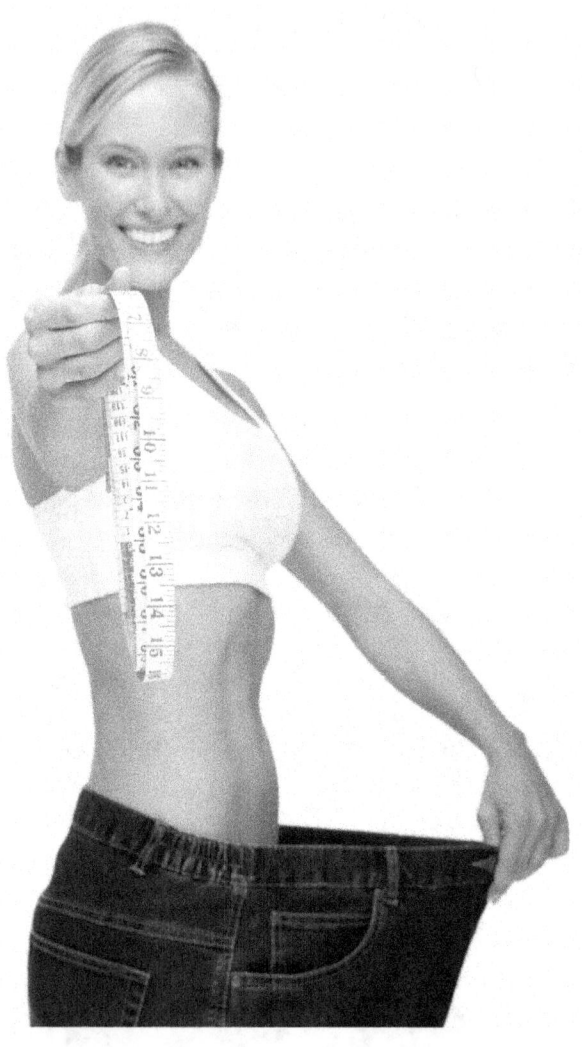

ABOUT THE AUTHOR

Victoria had a long career as a nutritionist; she lives in beautiful Santa Barbara, the city of her birth. Victoria struggled with her weight throughout her life until one day she discovered the power of detoxing and cleansing. An old century remedy a proven system to sweep out toxins that lead to weight gain, disease and energy swings.

www.ingramcontent.com/pod-product-compliance
Lightning Source LLC
Chambersburg PA
CBHW060505290526
45791CB00001B/273